Wanda Peresic, PT, DPT
Kansas City Kansas Community College
PTA Coordinator
Kansas City, KS

THE
ORTHOPEDIC
WORKBOOK
FOR PHYSICAL THERAPY

JONES AND BARTLETT PUBLISHERS
Sudbury, Massachusetts
BOSTON   TORONTO   LONDON   SINGAPORE

World Headquarters
Jones and Bartlett Publishers
40 Tall Pine Drive
Sudbury, MA 01776
978-443-5000
info@jbpub.com
www.jbpub.com

Jones and Bartlett Publishers Canada
6339 Ormindale Way
Mississauga, Ontario
L5V 1J2
CANADA

Jones and Bartlett Publishers International
Barb House, Barb Mews
London W6 7PA
UK

Jones and Bartlett's books and products are available through most bookstores and online booksellers. To contact
Jones and Bartlett Publishers directly, call 800-832-0034, fax 978-443-8000, or visit our website **www.jbpub.com**.

Substantial discounts on bulk quantities of Jones and Bartlett's publications are available to corporations,
professional associations, and other qualified organizations. For details and specific discount information,
contact the special sales department at Jones and Bartlett via the above contact information or send an
email to specialsales@jbpub.com.

The author has made every effort to ensure the accuracy of the information herein. However, appropriate information
sources should be consulted, especially for new or unfamiliar procedures. It is the responsibility of every practitioner
to evaluate the appropriateness of a particular opinion in the context of actual clinical situations and with due
considerations to new developments. The author(s) and publisher disclaim all responsibility for any liability, loss,
injury, or damage incurred as a consequence, directly or indirectly, of the use and application of any of the contents of
this volume.

6048

Production Credits
Executive Editor: David Cella
Production Director: Amy Rose
Production Assistant: Rachel Rossi
Editorial Assistant: Lisa Gordon
Associate Marketing Manager: Laura Kavigian
Manufacturing Buyer: Amy Bacus
Composition: Circle Graphics
Cover Design: Timothy Dziewit
Printing and Binding: Courier Stoughton
Cover Printing: Courier Stoughton

Printed in the United States of America
10 09 08 07 06   10 9 8 7 6 5 4 3 2 1

Dedication

This book is dedicated to my family and friends for supporting me during those late nights and time crunches. I would also like to thank my students for it is they who inspired me and taught me even more about physical therapy.

All images in this workbook were created with SmartDraw Software, which is available at: www.smartdraw.com.

In some instances, duplicate images have been provided to ensure that readers have the adequate space to effectively label diagrams.

Contents

Preface

This book was designed to help all physical therapist and physical therapist assistant students apply the basics of anatomy and progress through the evaluation, tests and measures, and interventions pursuant to the *Guide to Physical Therapy Practice.*

As an instructor in kinesiology and advanced treatment procedures, I have found that students cannot easily piece together, or have difficulty correlating the contents from one semester to another. This book is designed to help students put the pieces together, and be used throughout a curriculum, beginning in the first semester and continuing until graduation.

Chapter 1

AMERICAN PHYSICAL THERAPY ASSOCIATION'S (APTA) GUIDE TO PHYSICAL THERAPIST PRACTICE

Using the APTA's *Guide to Physical Therapist Practice*, answer the following questions:

PHYSICAL THERAPISTS

What education do physical therapists have?

According to the *Guide*, what does the physical therapist do?

Where do physical therapists practice?

Define the following: primary care, secondary care, and tertiary care.

According to the *Guide*, what is the definition of physical therapy? Does this definition differ from the State Practice Act definition?

List the five elements of the Patient/Client Management Model. Describe each.

PHYSICAL THERAPIST ASSISTANTS

What are physical therapist assistants?

What education do physical therapist assistants complete?

How do physical therapists differ from physical therapist assistants?

TESTS AND MEASURES

According to the *Guide*, tests and measures are used to get information needed for appropriate treatment. List five examples of tests and measures.

According to the *Guide*, define a measurement. Give three examples of a measurement.

According to the *Guide*, what would be the reasons that a physical therapist would use specific tests and measures?

Since this is a workbook, it is designed to break down general tests and measures as well as orthopedic tests. It should be made clear that orthopedic tests would fall under the test and measure category "Joint Integrity and Mobility." Also, please note that this workbook does not cover all of the orthopedic tests and measures, but the main ones that students will need to know.

INTERVENTIONS

Interventions are the treatment aspect of the management model. It is what is done on a daily basis with patients/clients. Give five examples of interventions.

What are the three components of an intervention described by the *Guide*?

PREFERRED PRACTICE PATTERNS

What are the practice patterns found in the "*Guide*"?

Chapter 2

GENERAL CONCEPTS

Kinesiology is the study of _____.

Orthopedics is the study of _____.

POSITIONS

When talking about positioning, there are various terms that are used. Define the following terms:

1. Anatomical position

2. Fundamental position

3. Supine

4. Prone

5. Sidelying

6. Recumbent

LOCATIONS

There are terms that are used in health and science to describe a location in relation to the anatomical position. Define the following terms:

1. Distal

2. Proximal

3. Cephalad

4. Caudal

5. Medial

6. Lateral

7. Superior

8. Inferior

9. Anterior

10. Posterior

11. Dorsal

12. Ventral

13. Plantar

14. Palmar

Fill in the blanks for the following statements:

1. The ankle is _____ to the knee.

2. The umbilicus is located on the _____ of the body.

3. The sacrum is more _____ than the occiput.

4. The thumb is more _____ than the little finger.

PLANES AND AXES ———————————————————————

There are three planes that divide the body. These include the Sagittal, Frontal, and Horizontal (Transverse).

Fill in the chart below for each of the planes.

Plane	Axis	Divides What Parts of the Body	Motions That Occur Within the Plane

Identify the three planes on the diagram below:

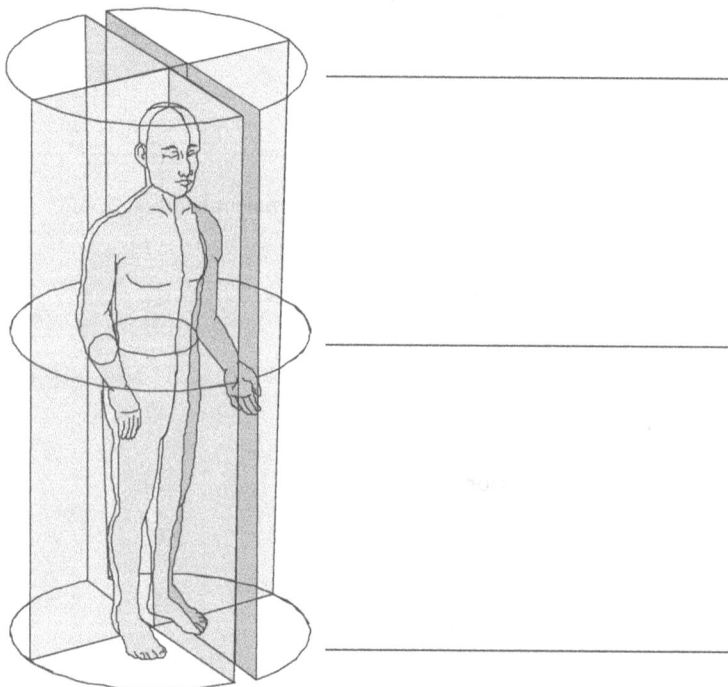

_____

_____

_____

Body in 3-D planes

JOINT MOTIONS

Describe the following motions:

1. Flexion

2. Extension

3. Abduction

4. Adduction

5. Internal Rotation

6. External Rotation

7. Supination

8. Pronation

9. Radial Deviation

10. Ulnar Deviation

11. Plantarflexion

12. Dorsiflexion

13. Lateral Flexion

14. Inversion

15. Eversion

16. Opposition

17. Circumduction

18. Protraction

19. Retraction

20. Protrusion

21. Retrusion

Complete the chart below:

Joint(s)	Motions Found Within the Joint
Shoulder	
Elbow	
Wrist	
Fingers	
Hip	
Knee	
Ankle	

Joint(s)	Motions Found Within the Joint
Toes	
Neck	
Temporo Mandibular Joint (TMJ)	
Thoracic-Lumbar Spine	

SKELETAL SYSTEM

The skeletal system's function is:

1.

2.

3.

4.

5.

There are two skeletal types found within the human body. Differentiate the two types.

1. Axial

2. Appendicular

The bones are made up of cancellous bone and compact bones. Identify each part of the bone below:

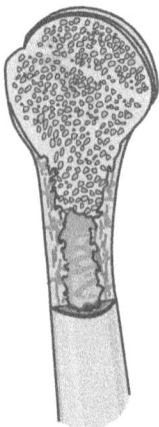

Bone parts

Identify the sections of the bone and define them: Epiphysis, Diaphysis, Metaphysis, and Periosteum.

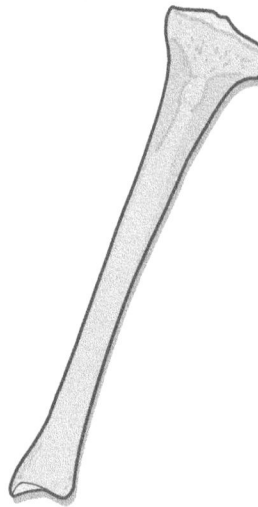

Bone sections

Shapes of Bones. Define the following terms:

1. Short

2. Long

3. Flat

4. Irregular

5. Sesmoid

Fill in the chart below:

Bones of the Body	Shape of Bone(s)
Skull	
Vertebra	
Ribs	
Sternum	
Pelvis	
Humerus	
Radius	
Ulna	
Carpals	
Metacarpals	
Phalanges	
Femur	
Tibia	
Fibula	
Tarsals	
Metatarsals	
Patella	

Identify the bones of the body on the skeletons below:

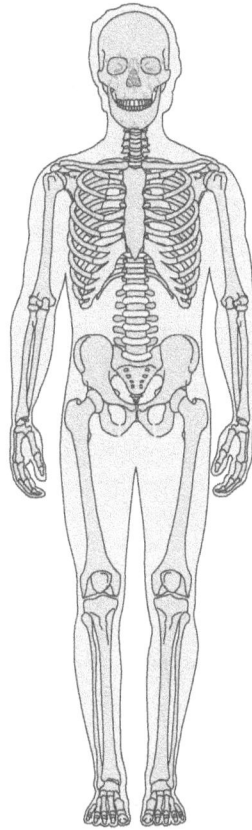

Anterior skeletal view

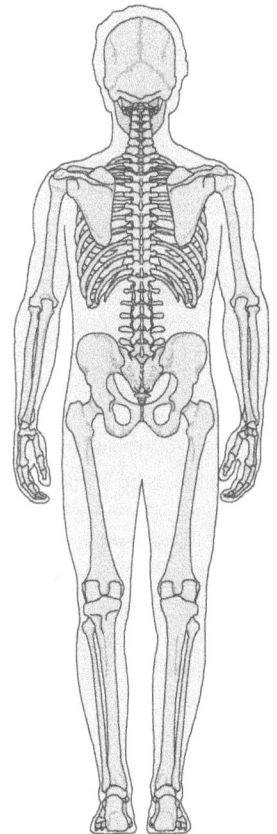

Posterior skeletal view

BONE MARKINGS/LANDMARKS ───────────────────────

Define the following terms:

1. Head

2. Condyle

3. Epicondyle

4. Tubercle, Tuberosity

5. Trochanter

6. Linea

7. Ridge

8. Neck

9. Groove

10. Foramen

11. Fossa

12. Process

Using your textbook, fill in the chart below:

Landmarks	Example	Bone Located on
Head	Humeral Head	Humerus
Condyle		
Epicondyle		
Tubercle, Tuberosity		
Trochanter		
Linea		
Ridge		
Neck		
Groove		
Foramen		
Fossa		
Process		

ARTICULAR SYSTEM

The function of the articular system is:

1.   4.

2.   5.

3.

There are several types (classifications) of joints in the body. Describe each type:

1. Fibrous (synarthrodial)   3. Synovial (diathrodial)

2. Cartilaginous (amphiarthrodial)

Synovial joints have different subclassifications. Describe each and include an example of each joint classification:

1. Nonaxial   3. Biaxial

2. Uniaxial   4. Triaxial

OPEN VERSUS CLOSED CHAIN

When the distal part of the extremity moves on the proximal part of the extremity, this is called
_____.

When the distal part of the extremity is fixed and the proximal part of the extremity moves on distal end, this is called _____.

Give an example:

Give an example:

JOINT MOTION

Define arthrokinematics:

When a bone moves on another bone, motion occurs. Depending on the type of the joint, roll, glide/slide, and spin motions can occur within the joint. Describe each joint motion, then give an example within the body and outside of the body.

1. Roll   3. Spin

2. Glide (slide)

The bones are made up of either a convex or a concave surface. A convex surface is the part of a bone that is protruding away from midline. A concave surface is when the part of the bone is caved toward midline of the bone. Fill in the chart below.

Joint	First Bone That Forms the Joint	Convex or Concave	Second Bone That Forms the Joint	Convex or Concave	In Open Chain, Describe the Motion	In Closed Chain, Describe the Motion
Shoulder	Scapula	Concave	Humerus	Convex	Roll and Glide are Opposite	Roll and Glide are the Same
Elbow						
Wrist						
Fingers						
Hip						
Knee						
Ankle						
Toes						
Neck						
TMJ						
Thoracic-Lumbar Spine						

Osteokinematics

Osteokinematics is defined as the range of motion a joint has. Each joint's normal range of motion will be reviewed in its respective chapter.

Define each term as it pertains to range of motion. Document what is seen when a patient/client is observed with each one.

1. Hypomobility

2. Hypermobility

3. Contracture

Muscular System

Endomysium surrounds each muscle. Muscles are made up of sections called fasciculi. Fasciculi are surrounded by connective tissue called perimysium. Fasciculi are made up of many muscle fibers. Each muscle fiber is surrounded by endomysium. Myofibrils are found within each fiber. Myofibrils are made up of myofilaments. These myofilaments are called actin and myosin.

Draw the muscle structure and the sections below:

Myofilaments, actin and myosin, are responsible for the contraction of a muscle. Sarcomeres are found within the myofilament. Below is a sarcomere. Identify the following: Z lines, M band, I band, H zone, A band, actin and myosin.

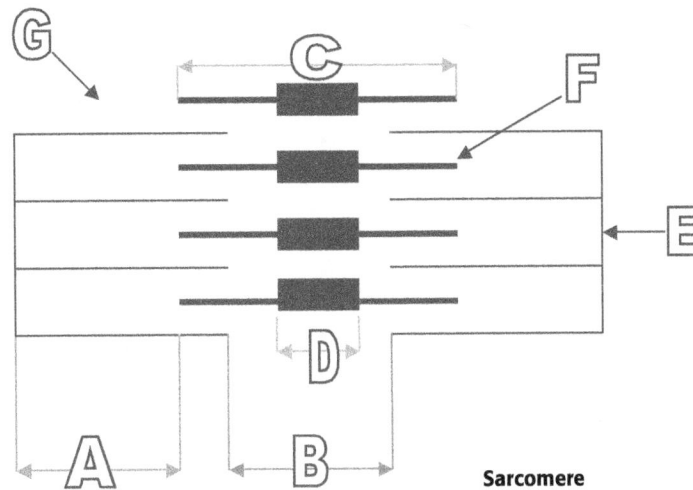

Sarcomere

Describe each term:

1. A band

2. H zone

3. I band

4. M band

5. Z lines

Compare and contrast actin and myosin:

Define the following and the role that each plays in the muscle:

1. Sharkey's Fibers

2. Golgi Tendon Organs

3. Muscle Spindle

Normally, muscles move from the origin to the insertion. Define the following terms:

1. Origin

2. Insertion

Muscles contract concentrically, eccentrically or isometrically. Define the following terms:

1. Concentric

2. Eccentric

3. Isometric

You are flexing your elbow. What group of muscles (elbow flexors versus elbow extensors) will be working concentrically?

You are doing a squat. You are slowly allowing your knees to bend. What group of muscles is working eccentrically?

What contraction has the most force generated?

Muscles have various arrangements of their fibers. Parallel fibers run along the long axis of the muscle. Oblique fibers run at an angle. Parallel muscle fibers can be a strap muscle, fusiform muscle, rhomboidal muscle or triangular. Oblique muscle fibers can be unipennate, bipennate, or multipennate. Draw the following fiber arrangements:

1. Fusiform

Give an example of a fusiform muscle:

2. Strap

Give an example of a strap muscle:

3. Rhomboidal

Give an example of a rhomboidal muscle:

4. Unipennate

Give an example of an unipennate muscle:

5. Bipennate

Give an example of a bipennate muscle:

6. Multipennate

Give an example of a multipennate muscle:

Compare parallel and oblique muscle fibers:

Length Tension Relationship

The muscle has characteristics that make it functional. These include irritability, extensibility, contractility, and elasticity. Explain the role of each of the following:

Irritability:

Extensibility:

Contractility:

Elasticity:

Generally, if a person is in the anatomical position:

1. The muscles on the anterior surface of the body will perform what motion?

2. The muscles on the posterior surface of the body will perform what motion?

3. The muscles on the lateral surface of the body will perform what motion?

4. The muscles on the medial surface of the body will perform what motion?

Define the following terms:

1. Agonist

2. Antagonist

3. Synergist

4. Active Insufficiency

5. Passive Insufficiency

6. Tenodesis

7. Concentric Contraction

8. Eccentric Contraction

9. Isometric Contraction

Nervous System

The nerve cells are made up of the axon, the dendrite, and the cell body. Label the components in the following nerve cell. Describe the functions of each component.

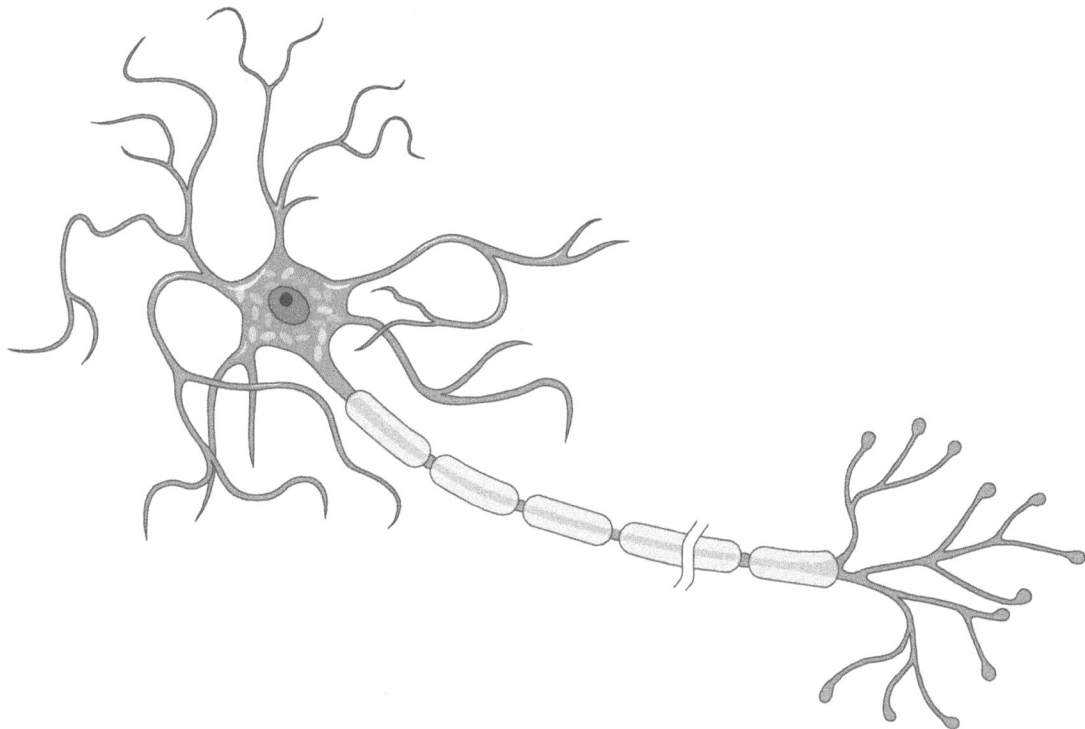

Nerve cell

The nervous system is made up of the central nervous system and the peripheral nervous system. Explain the difference between the two. If a patient sustains an injury to the central nervous system, how would it be different than if the patient sustained an injury to the peripheral nervous system?

What is the function of the efferent (motor) nerve and the afferent (sensory) nerve?

The reflex arc consists of a receptor, afferent nerve, center, efferent nerve, and the effector. Identify each on the diagram below.

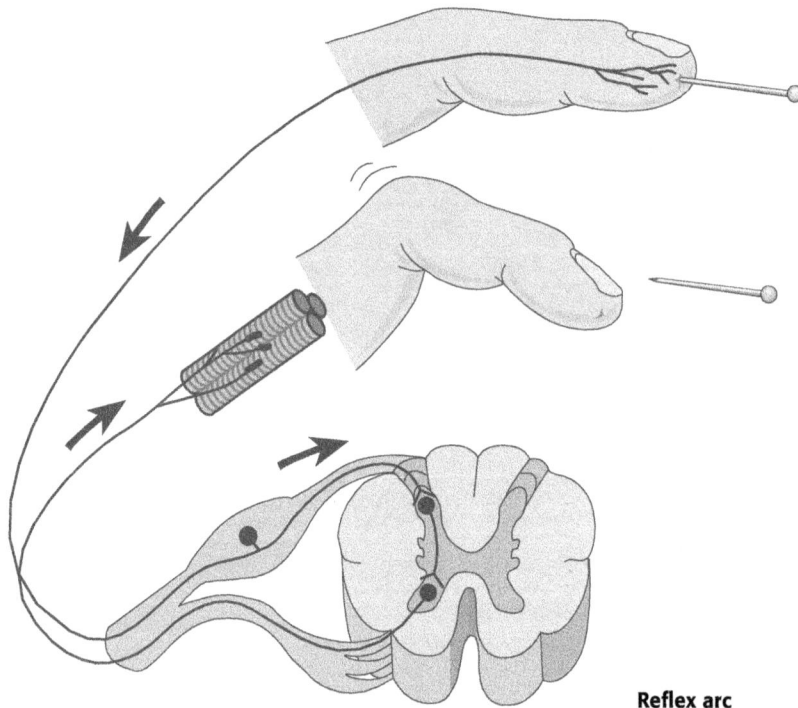

Reflex arc

Chapter 3

Biomechanics

Define the following terms:

1. Biomechanics

2. Kinetics

3. Kinematics

Give an anatomical and a nonanatomical example of each of the following descriptors of kinematics:

Rotatory:

　Anatomical:

　Nonanatomical:

Translatory:

　Anatomical:

　Nonanatomical:

Curvilinear:

　Anatomical:

　Nonanatomical:

Forces: Force is the effect that one object has on another by direct contact. This can be described as a push or pull. There are basically two types of forces that will be addressed: internal and external. In the space below, give three examples of external and internal forces that deal with the human body.

Vectors describe the magnitude of force applied to an object, the area on an object in which it is being acted on, and the action and direction the force is being exerted.

In the diagram below, draw a vector that shows the action and the direction the weight has on the lifter.

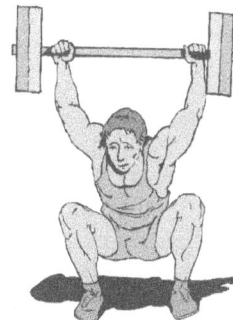

What is the center of gravity in the human body when standing in the anatomical position?

How will the center of gravity change when a person bends forward?

NEWTON'S LAWS

1. Newton's Law of Inertia (Newton's 1st Law) states that an object will remain at rest or in equilibrium until an unbalanced force is placed against the object.

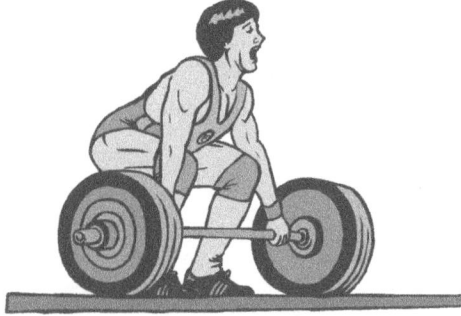

In the diagram above, assume that the weights (totaling 100 pounds) are resting quietly on the floor. Using vectors show Newton's 1st Law.

2. Newton's Law of Acceleration (Newton's 2nd Law) states that the acceleration of an object is proportional to the unequal forces placed upon it and is inversely proportional to the weight (mass) of that object. The equation for acceleration is: a (acceleration) = F (force)/m (mass). For example, the greater the internal force of the quadriceps and hip flexors a football kicker has, the more acceleration will be placed on the leg in order to kick the ball. Consider two kickers, one being 90 pounds and the other being 190 pounds. The kicker who is 190 pounds will have a greater acceleration because the force needed to move the weight of the leg is greater.

3. Newton's Law of Reaction (Newton's 3rd Law) states that for every action there is an equal and opposite reaction. This means that if object A applies a force to a weight (object B), the weight must apply the same force against object A. If the above weightlifter is to lift 100 pounds, simplistically, the weight is applying 100 pounds against the weightlifter. Keep in mind that the effect of gravity on the weight is not being considered.

What happens if one force is more than the other?

Lever Systems: Looking inside the body and the muscle system, it can be seen that muscles use a pulley-like mechanism to gain the appropriate pull (contraction) on the muscle. Besides the pulley mechanism, the anatomical composition of our muscles also uses a lever system between the muscles and the skeletal system.

There are three lever systems that are used in the body: 1st class lever, 2nd class lever, and 3rd class lever.

Draw each of the levers found in the body and give an anatomical and nonanatomical example of each.

1. 1st class lever

2. 2nd class lever

3. 3rd class lever

The stress/strain curve is used to demonstrate the amount of stress that is applied to a tissue before deformation occurs. If the load is progressive, there will be a point in time where the tissue will fail or break. Draw the stress/strain curve on the tissues mentioned below.

1. Bone:

2. Tendon:

3. Ligaments:

4. Cartilage:

Chapter 4

SHOULDER

ANATOMY ——————————————————————————————————

Skeletal System:

1. Scapula

2. Clavicle

3. Sternum

4. Humerus

Label the above bones on the diagram below:

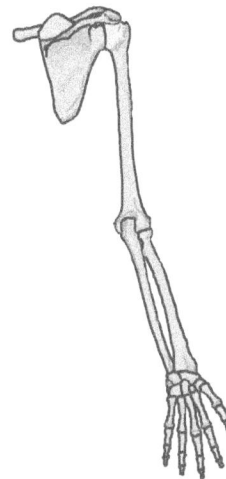

Posterior view of right arm and shoulder

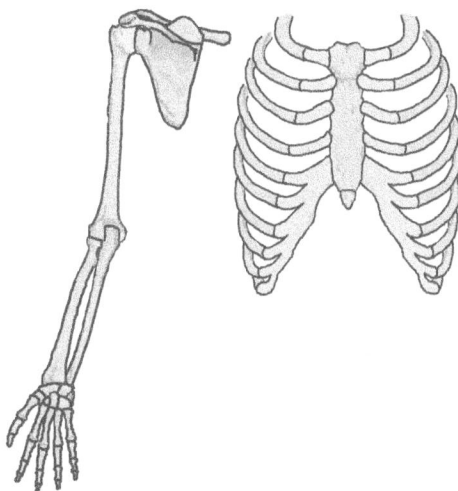

Anterior view of rib cage with right arm

Label the following bony landmarks on the diagram above:

Greater Tuberosity	Lesser Tuberosity
Bicipital Groove	Head of the Humerus
Surgical Neck	Anatomical Neck
Humeral Medial Condyle	Humeral Lateral Condyle
Supraspinous Fossa	Infraspinous Fossa
Subscapular Fossa	Glenoid Fossa
Spine of Scapula	Root of the Spine
Axillary Border (Lateral Border)	Vertebral Border (Medial Border)
Acromion	Coracoid Process
Inferior Angle	Superior Angle
Manubrium	Body
Xiphoid Process	Sternal End of Clavicle
Acromial End of Clavicle	Shaft of Clavicle

Muscular System:

Muscles anterior of the shoulder:

1. Coracobrachialis

2. Biceps Brachii

3. Pectoralis Major

4. Pectoralis Minor

5. Subclavius

6. Serratus Anterior

7. Anterior Deltoid

8. Subscapularis

Draw the above muscles on the diagrams below:

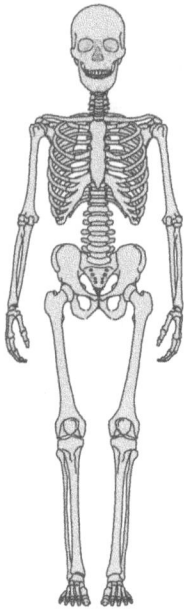

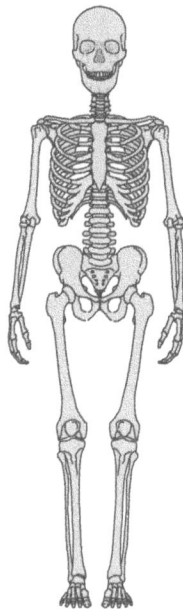

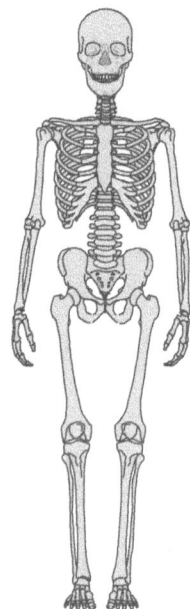

Anterior skeletal views

Muscles posterior of the shoulder:

1. Triceps

2. Posterior Deltoid

3. Supraspinatus

4. Infraspinatus

5. Teres Major

6. Teres Minor

7. Rhomboid Major

8. Rhomboid Minor

9. Upper Trapezius

10. Middle Trapezius

11. Lower Trapezius

12. Latissimus Dorsi

13. Levator Scapula

Draw the muscles on the diagrams below:

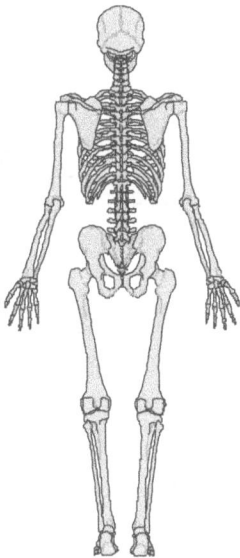

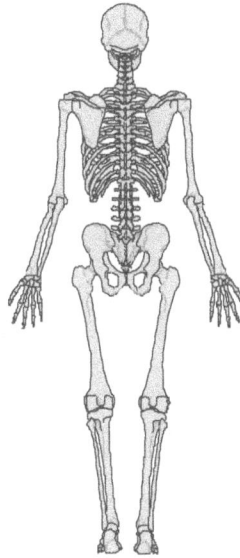

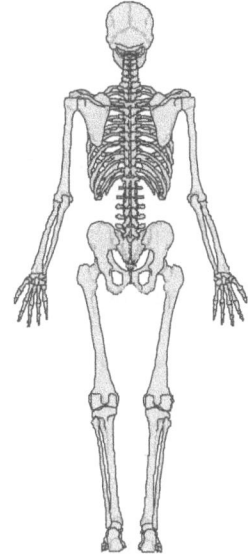

Posterior skeletal views

Muscles lateral of the shoulder:

1. Middle Deltoid

Fill in the blanks in the charts below:

Flexors of the Shoulder	Origin	Insertion	Action	Innervation of the Muscle	Nerve Root Level
Coracobrachialis					
Anterior Deltoid					
Pectoralis Major					
Biceps Brachii					

Extensors of the Shoulder	Origin	Insertion	Action	Innervation of the Muscle	Nerve Root Level
Latissimus Dorsi					
Teres Major					
Pectoralis Major					
Posterior Deltoid					
Infraspinatus					
Teres Minor					
Triceps Brachii					

Abductors of the Shoulder	Origin	Insertion	Action	Innervation of the Muscle	Nerve Root Level
Middle Deltoid					
Supraspinatus					

Adductors of the Shoulder	Origin	Insertion	Action	Innervation of the Muscle	Nerve Root Level
Pectoralis Major					
Latissimus Dorsi					
Teres Major					
Coracobrachialis					

External Rotators of the Shoulder	Origin	Insertion	Action	Innervation of the Muscle	Nerve Root Level
Infraspinatus					
Teres Minor					
Posterior Deltoid					

Internal Rotators of the Shoulder	Origin	Insertion	Action	Innervation of the Muscle	Nerve Root Level
Anterior Deltoid					
Pectoralis Major					
Subscapularis					
Teres Major					
Latissimus Dorsi					

Scapular Elevators	Origin	Insertion	Action	Innervation of the Muscle	Nerve Root Level
Upper Trapezius					
Levator Scapula					

Scapular Depressors	Origin	Insertion	Action	Innervation of the Muscle	Nerve Root Level
Pectoralis Major					
Lower Trapezius					

Scapular Protractors	Origin	Insertion	Action	Innervation of the Muscle	Nerve Root Level
Pectoralis Minor					
Serratus Anterior					

Scapular Retractors	Origin	Insertion	Action	Innervation of the Muscle	Nerve Root Level
Middle Trapezius					
Rhomboid					

Scapular Upward Rotators	Origin	Insertion	Action	Innervation of the Muscle	Nerve Root Level
Upper Trapezius					
Lower Trapezius					
Serratus Anterior					

Scapular Downward Rotators	Origin	Insertion	Action	Innervation of the Muscle	Nerve Root Level
Levator Scapula					
Rhomboids					
Pectoralis Major					

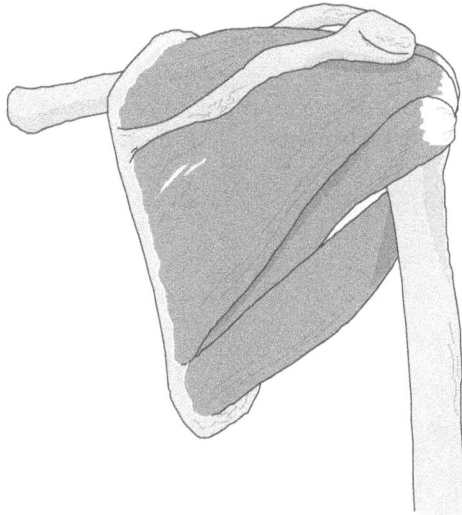

Shoulder with muscles

On the diagrams below, color the area(s) that are innervated by the nerves mentioned in the charts previous:

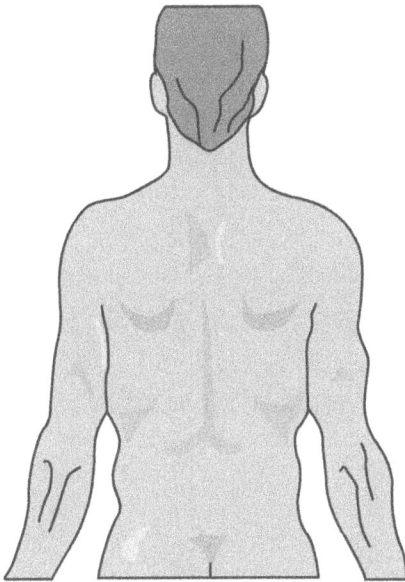

Posterior view of male trunk

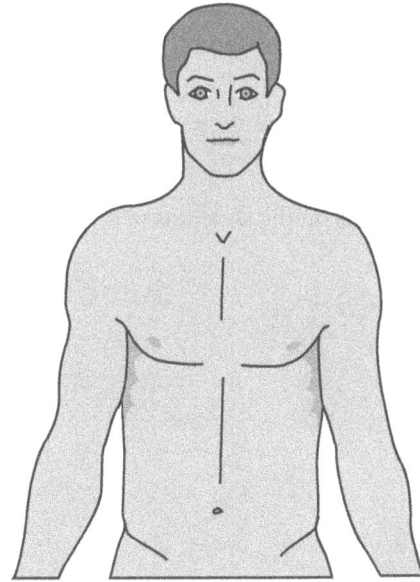

Anterior view of male trunk

CONNECTIVE TISSUE

The main ligaments of the shoulder include:

1. Superior, Middle, and Inferior Glenohumeral Ligament

2. Coracohumeral Ligament

3. Interclavicular Ligament

4. Costoclavicular Ligament

5. Anterior Sternoclavicular Ligament

6. Posterior Sternoclavicular Ligament

7. Coracoclavicular Ligament

8. Acromioclavicular Ligament

9. Coracoacromial Ligament

Fill in the blanks in the chart below:

Ligaments	Stabilizes What Joint	Attachments	Function	Clinical Presentation When Laxity Is Present
Superior, Middle, and Inferior Glenohumeral				
Coracohumeral				
Interclavicular				
Costoclavicular				
Anterior Sternoclavicular				
Posterior Sternoclavicular				
Coracoclavicular				
Acromioclavicular				
Coracoacromial				

Draw the ligaments on the skeletons of the arm and ribcage below:

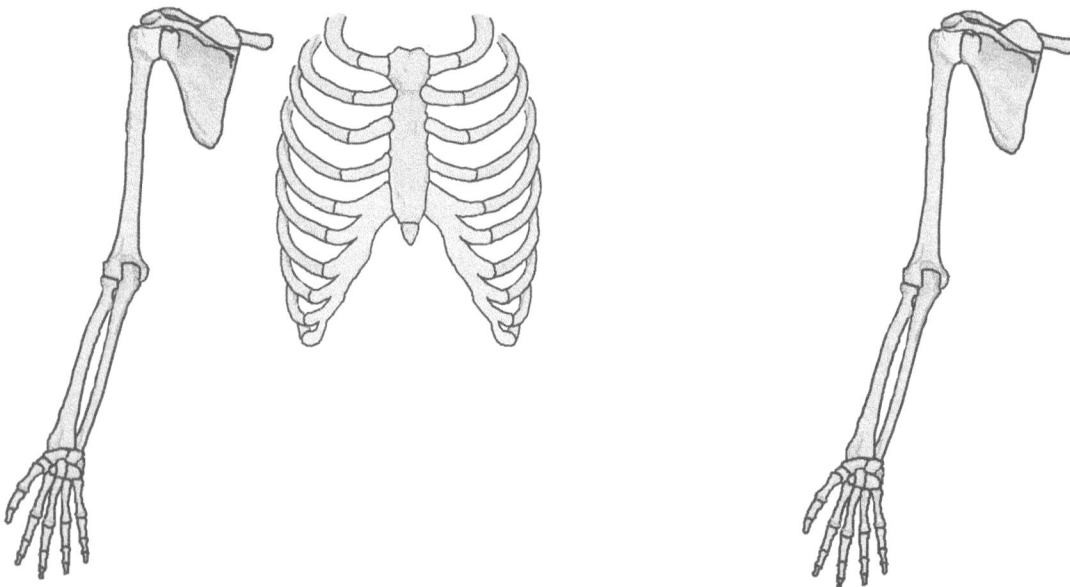

BURSA

There are numerous bursa found around the elbow. Place the positions of the following bursa on the diagram above:

1. Subscapular

2. Subacromial

3. Subcoracoid

ARTHROKINEMATICS

What is the closed pack position of the shoulder?

What is the loose packed position of the shoulder?

Fill in the correct range of motion measurements:

Shoulder Flexion   _____

Shoulder Extension   _____

Shoulder Internal Rotation   _____

Shoulder External Rotation   _____

Shoulder Abduction   _____

Shoulder Adduction   _____

Scapular Protraction   _____

Scapular Retraction   _____

Glenohumeral Flexion   _____

Glenohumeral Abduction   _____

Scapulohumeral Flexion   _____

Scapulohumeral Abduction   _____

If a person is sitting in a chair and with their shoulders at 90 degrees of flexion and then the person horizontally abducts their shoulders, is the action moving convex on concave or concave on convex? What direction is the roll? The glide?

Brachial Plexus

In order to fully understand the innervation of the upper extremity, you must have a concept of how the nerves enter the upper extremity from the cervical spine. Draw the brachial plexus from the diagram below:

| C1 |
| C2 |
| C3 |
| C4 |
| C5 |
| C6 |
| C7 |
| C8 |
| T1 |

Commonly Treated Diagnoses of the Shoulder Complex

1. Bursitis

2. Supraspinatus Tendonitis

3. Bicipital Tendonitis

4. Muscle Strain

5. Fractures

6. Total Shoulder Replacement

7. Arthritis

8. Dislocations

9. Rotator Cuff Tear

10. Labral Injuries

11. Impingement

12. Acromioclavicular Ligament Injuries

Using the *Guide* and your orthopedic textbook, fill in the chart below for the pathologies noted:

Pathology	Tissues Affected	Pathophysiology	Clinical Presentations	Preferred Practice Pattern
Bursitis				
Supraspinatus Tendonitis				
Bicipital Tendonitis				
Muscle Strain				
Fractures				
Total Shoulder Replacement				
Arthritis				
Dislocations				
Rotator Cuff Tear				
Labral Injuries				
Impingement				
Acromioclavicular Ligament Injuries				

Common Orthopedic Tests of the Shoulder

1. Apprehension (Crank) Test

2. Fulcrum Test

3. Anterior Drawer Test

4. Posterior Drawer Test

5. Sulcus Test

6. Clunk Test

7. Speed's Test

8. Yergason's Test

9. Empty Can Test

10. Drop Arm Test

11. Neer's Impingement Test

12. Roo's Test

13. Adson's Test

14. Allen's Test

Orthopedic Tests	Procedure for Testing	Characteristics of a Positive Outcome	Anatomical Structures Being Tested
Apprehension (Crank) Test			
Fulcrum Test			
Anterior Drawer Test			
Posterior Drawer Test			
Sulcus Test			
Clunk Test			
Speed's Test			
Yergason's Test			
Empty Can Test			
Drop Arm Test			
Neer's Test			
Roo's Test			
Adson's Test			
Allen's Test			

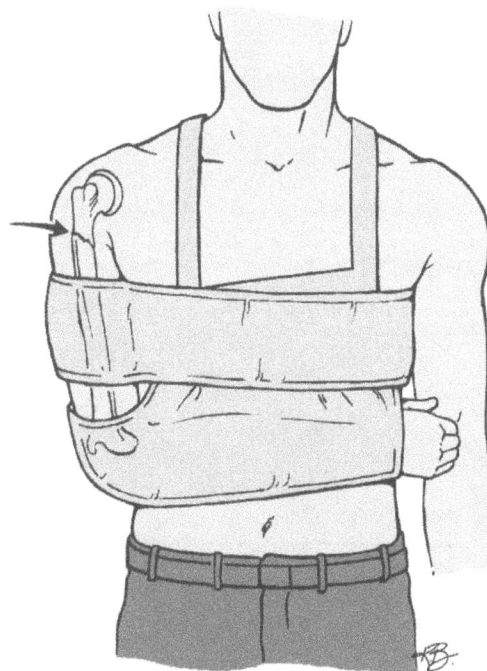

Torso with support wrap for fracture

OTHER TESTS AND MEASURES PERFORMED ON THE SHOULDER

Pathology	Tests and Measures	What Is the Test and Measure Testing?	Possible Abnormal Findings
Bursitis			
Supraspinatus Tendonitis			
Bicipital Tendonitis			
Muscle Strain			
Fractures			
Total Shoulder Arthroplasty			
Rotator Cuff Tear			
Arthritis			
Dislocations			
Labral Injuries			
Impingement			
Ligamentous Injuries			

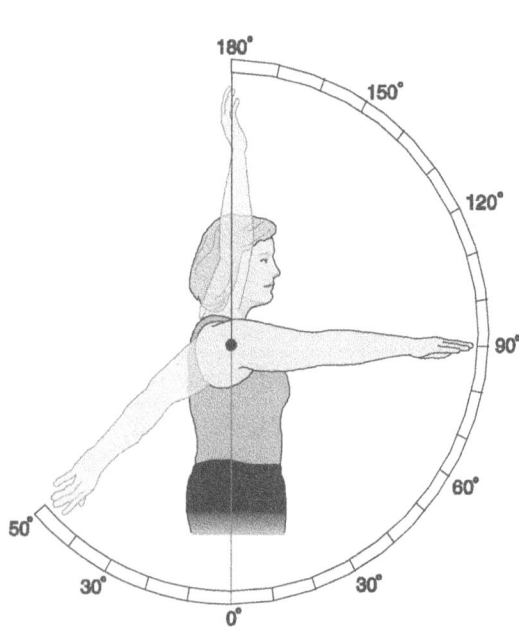

Shoulder arc, right side view

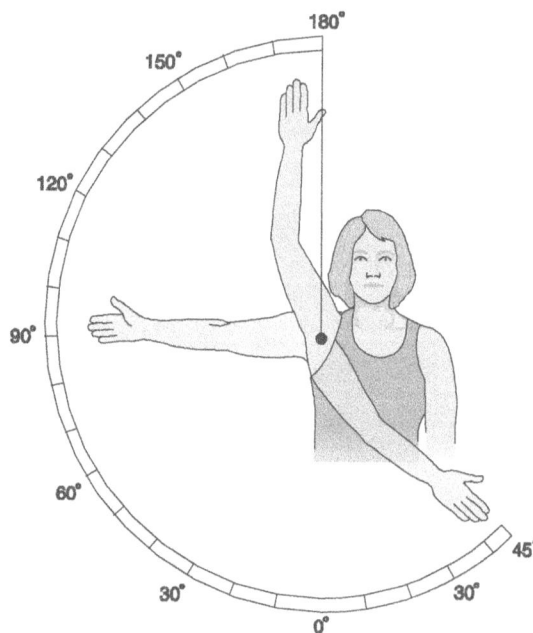

Shoulder arc, anterior view

INTERVENTIONS

Pathology	Interventions	Indications for Interventions	Goals of Intervention	Contraindications for Interventions	Settings for Interventions
Bursitis					
Supraspinatus Tendonitis					
Bicipital Tendonitis					
Muscle Strain					
Fractures					
Total Shoulder Arthroplasty					
Arthritis					
Dislocations					
Rotator Cuff Tear					
Labral Injuries					
Impingement Syndrome					
Anterior Cruciate Ligament Injury					

Chapter 5

ELBOW

ANATOMY

Skeletal System:

1. Humerus

2. Ulna
   a. The true elbow joint is made up of the humerus and the ulna.

3. Humerus

Label the following bones on the diagrams below:

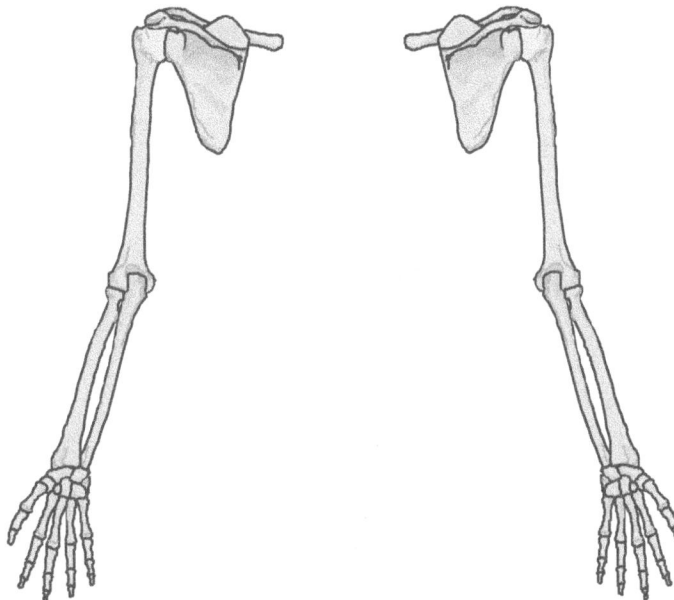

Right and left arm skeletal structures

Label the following bony landmarks on the diagram above:

Humeral Medial Condyle and
  Epicondyle
Humeral Lateral Condyle
  and Epicondyle

Radial Fossa
Capitulum
Radial Head
Olecranon Process

Olecranon Fossa
Coronoid Process
Styloid Process
  of the Radius

Trochlea
Coronoid Fossa
Styloid Process
  of the Ulna

Muscular System:

Muscles anterior of the elbow:

1. Biceps Brachii

2. Brachialis

3. Brachioradialis

4. Pronator Teres

5. Pronator Quadratus

6. Supinator

Draw the above muscles on the diagrams below:

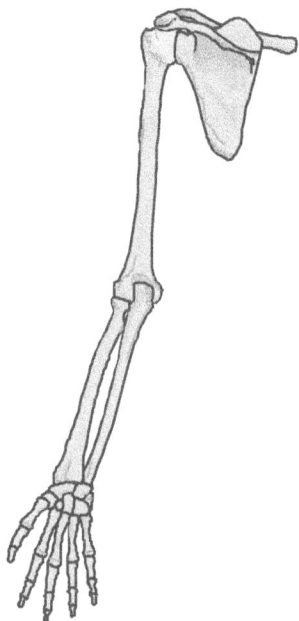

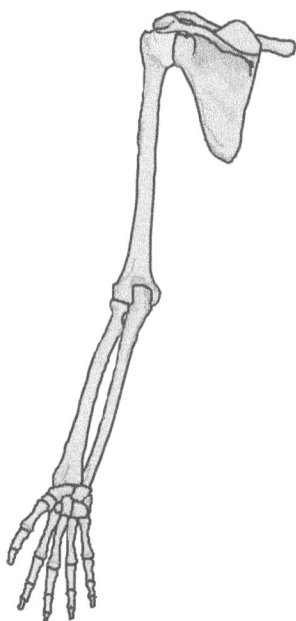

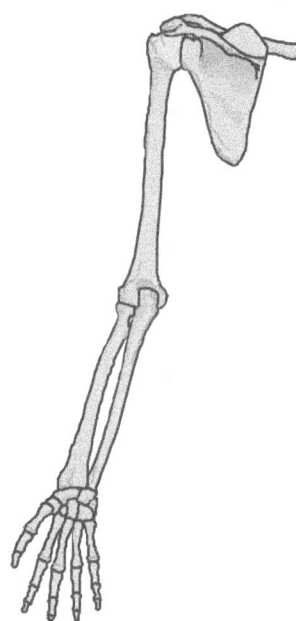

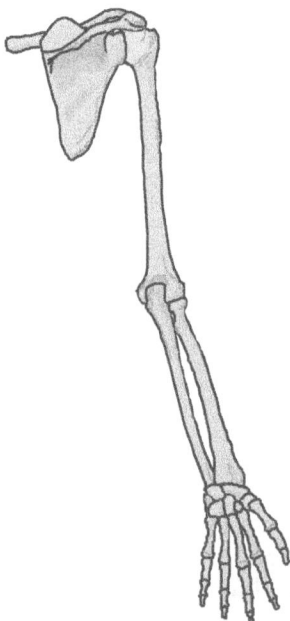

Muscles posterior of the elbow:

1. Triceps Brachii

2. Anconeus

Draw the muscles on the diagram below:

Fill in the blanks of the charts below:

Flexors of the Elbow	Origin	Insertion	Action	Innervation of the Muscle	Nerve Root Level
Biceps Brachii					
Brachialis					
Brachioradialis					

Extensors of the Elbow	Origin	Insertion	Action	Innervation of the Muscle	Nerve Root Level
Triceps Brachii					
Anconeus					

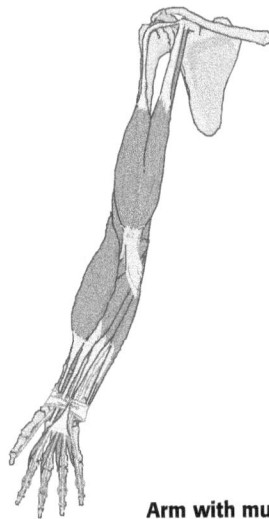

Arm with musculature

Supinators of the Elbow	Origin	Insertion	Action	Innervation of the Muscle	Nerve Root Level
Biceps Brachii					
Supinator					

Pronators of the Elbow	Origin	Insertion	Action	Innervation of the Muscle	Nerve Root Level
Pronator Teres					
Pronator Quadratus					

On the diagrams below, color the area(s) that are innervated by the nerves mentioned above:

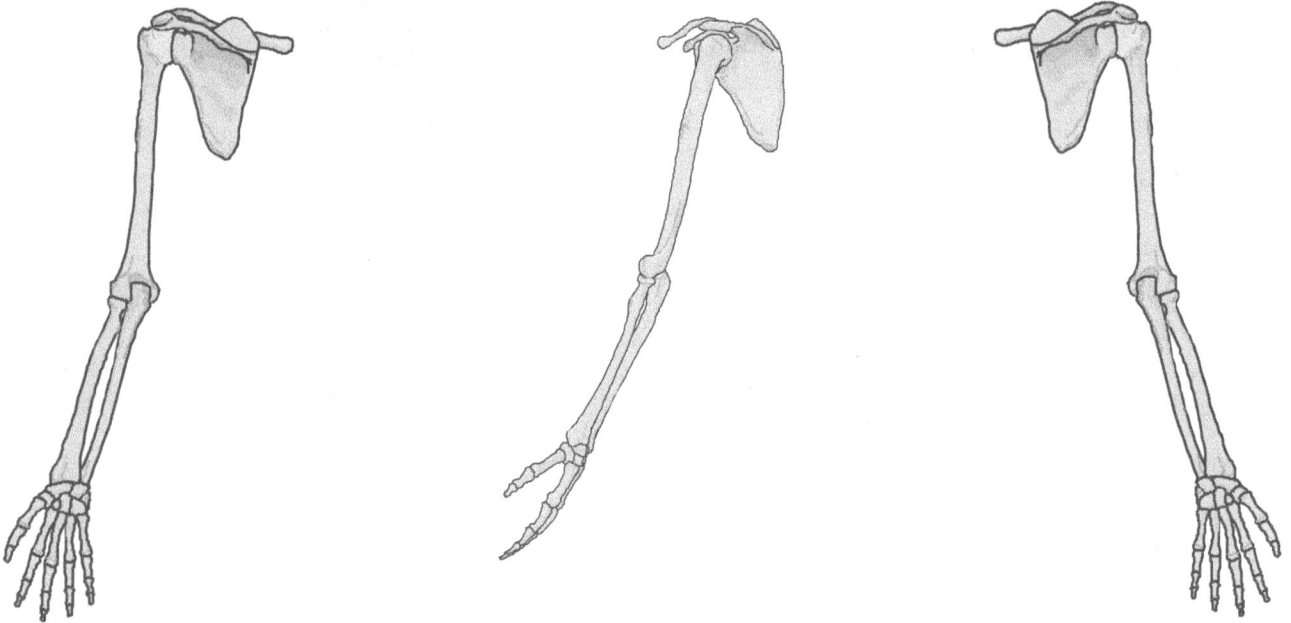

Anterior, Lateral and Posterior views of skeletal structure of arm

CONNECTIVE TISSUE ——————————————————————————————————

The main ligaments of the elbow include:

1. Annular Ligament

2. Medial Collateral Ligament

3. Lateral Collateral Ligament

4. Interosseus Membrane

5. Quadrate Ligament

Fill in the blanks in the chart below:

Ligaments	Stabilizes What Joint	Location	Function	Clinical Presentation When Laxity Is Present
Annular				
Medial Collateral				
Lateral Collateral				
Interosseus Membrane				
Quadrate Ligament				

Draw the Olecranon Bursa on the diagram below:

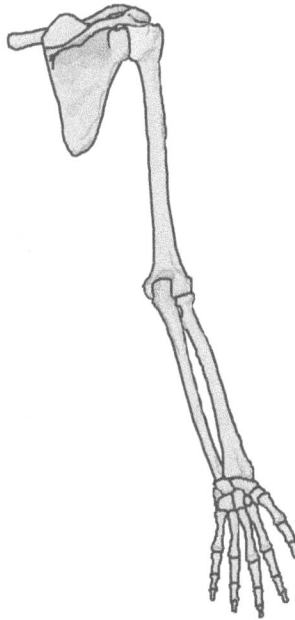

ARTHROKINEMATICS ───────────────────────────────

What is the closed pack position of the elbow?

What is the carrying angle? What is the normal carrying angle for women? For men?

What is the loose pack position of the elbow?

Fill in the correct range of motion measurements:

Elbow Flexion _____

Elbow Extension _____

Supination _____

Pronation _____

If you are turning the door handle with your right arm to the right, are you moving convex on concave or concave on convex?

If you do a bicep curl, are you moving convex on concave or concave on convex? What direction is the roll? The glide?

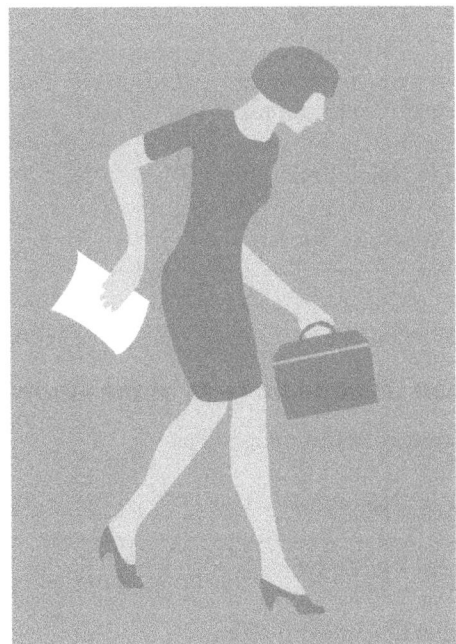

COMMON TREATED DIAGNOSIS OF THE ELBOW JOINT ——————————

1. Lateral Epicondylitis

2. Medial Epicondylitis

3. Muscle Strain

4. Fractures

5. Total Joint Replacement

6. Radial Dislocations

7. Ulnar Dislocations

8. Arthritis

9. Ulnar Nerve Entrapment

10. Median Nerve Entrapment

11. Olecranon Bursitis

Using the *Guide* and your orthopedic textbook, fill in the chart below for the pathologies:

Pathology	Tissues Affected	Pathophysiology	Clinical Presentations	Preferred Practice Pattern
Lateral Epicondylitis				
Medial Epicondylitis				
Muscle Strain				
Fractures				
Total Joint Replacement				
Radial Dislocations				
Ulnar Dislocations				
Arthritis				
Ulnar Nerve Entrapment				
Median Nerve Entrapment				
Olecranon Bursitis				

Common Orthopedic Tests of the Elbow

1. Ligamentous Instability Test

2. Lateral Epicondylitis Test 1

3. Lateral Epicondylitis Test 2

4. Medial Epicondylitis Test

5. Tinel's Sign

Orthopedic Test	Procedure for Testing	Characteristics of a Positive Outcome	Anatomical Structures Being Tested
Ligamentous Instability Test			
Lateral Epicondylitis Test 1			
Lateral Epicondylitis Test 2			
Medial Epicondylitis Test			
Tinel's Sign			

OTHER TESTS AND MEASURES PERFORMED ON THE ELBOW

Pathology	Tests and Measures	What Is the Test and Measure Testing?	Possible Abnormal Findings
Lateral Epicondylitis			
Medial Epicondylitis			
Muscle Strain			
Fractures			
Total Joint Replacement			
Radial Dislocations			
Ulnar Dislocations			
Arthritis			
Ulnar Nerve Entrapment			
Median Nerve Entrapment			
Olecranon Bursitis			

INTERVENTIONS

Pathology	Interventions	Indications for Intervention	Goals for the Intervention	Contraindications of the Intervention	Settings for Intervention
Example	Ultrasound	Increase in pain, edema, and increase in inflammatory response.	To decrease pain, decrease inflammatory response, and increase circulation to facilitate healing.	Pacemakers, cancer, plastic implants, pregnancy, joint cement, and decreased sensation and mentation.	Will use a pulsed ultrasound 1 MHz at 2.0 w/cm^2 at 100% duty cycle × 10 minutes. Phonophoresis may be beneficial as well.
Lateral Epicondylitis					
Medial Epicondylitis					
Muscle Strain					
Fractures					
Total Joint Replacement					
Radial Dislocations					
Ulnar Dislocations					
Arthritis					
Ulnar Nerve Entrapment					
Median Nerve Entrapment					
Olecranon Bursitis					

Chapter 6

WRIST AND HAND

ANATOMY

Skeletal System:

1. Radius
2. Ulna
3. Scaphoid
4. Triquetrium
5. Lunate
6. Pisiform

7. Hamate
8. Trapezoid
9. Trapezium
10. Capitate
11. Metacarpals
12. Phalanges

Label the above bones on the diagram below:

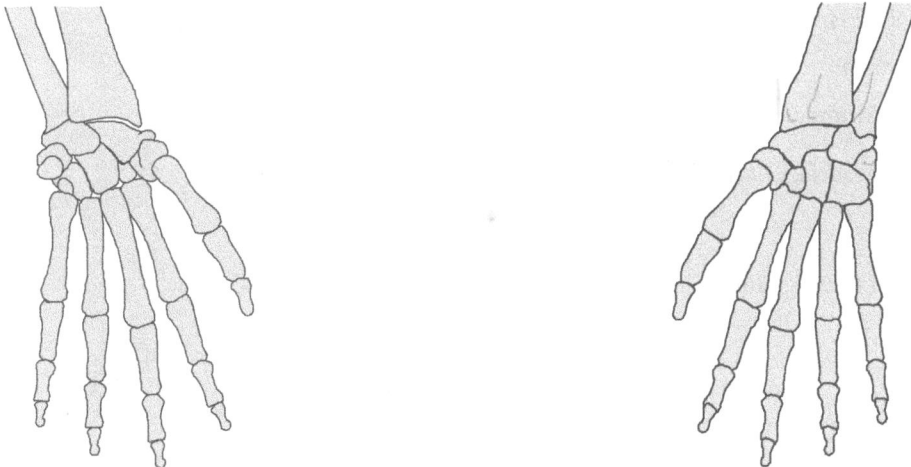

Skeletal structure of wrists and hands, right and left views

Label the following bony landmarks on the diagram above, right:

1. Metacarpal Head
2. Metacarpal Base
3. Metacarpal Shaft
4. Phalangeal Head

5. Phalangeal Base
6. Phalangeal Shaft
7. Radial Styloid Process
8. Ulnar Styloid Process

Muscular System:

Muscles of the anterior surface of the wrist and forearm:

1. Palmaris Longus
2. Flexor Carpi Radialis
3. Flexor Carpi Ulnaris

4. Flexor Digitorum Superficialis
5. Flexor Digitorum Profundus
6. Flexor Pollicis Longus

Draw the above muscles on the diagrams below:

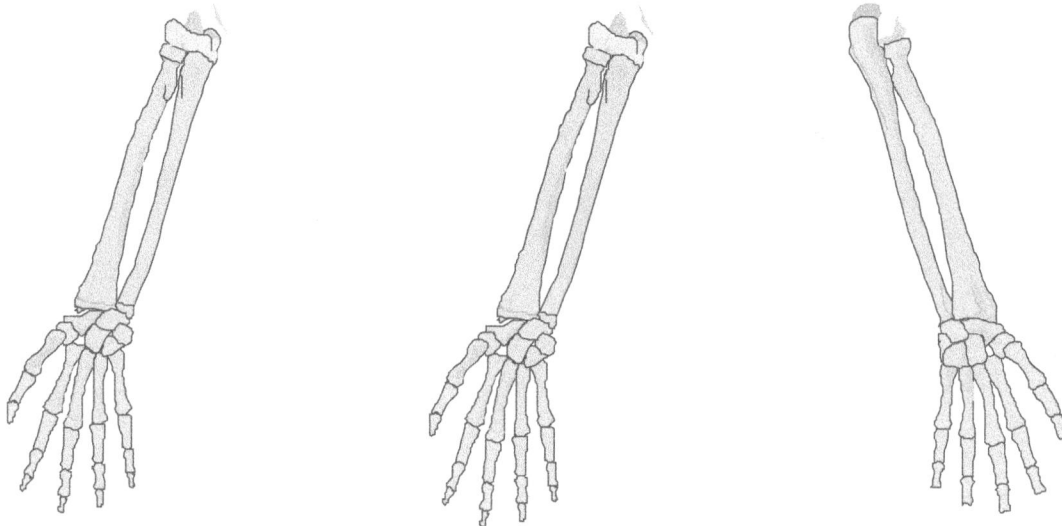

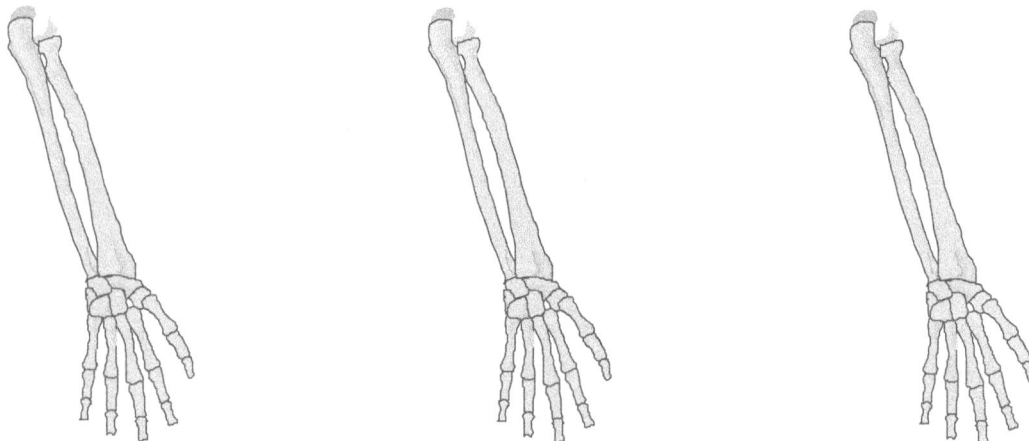

Muscles on the posterior surface of the wrist and forearm:

1. Extensor Carpi Radialis Brevis
2. Extensor Carpi Radialis Longus
3. Extensor Carpi Ulnaris
4. Extensor Digitorum
5. Extensor Digiti Minimi

6. Extensor Indicis
7. Abductor Pollicis Longus
8. Extensor Pollicis Brevis
9. Extensor Pollicis Longus

Muscles on the lateral surface of the forearm:

1. Supinator

Draw the muscles on the diagrams below:

Muscles on the anterior surface of the hand:

1. Abductor Pollicis Brevis

2. Adductor Pollicis

3. Flexor Pollicis Brevis

4. Flexor Digiti Minimi

5. Opponens Pollicis

6. Opponens Digiti Minimi

7. Abductor Digiti Minimi

8. Palmar Interossei

9. Lumbricals

Draw the above muscles on the diagrams below:

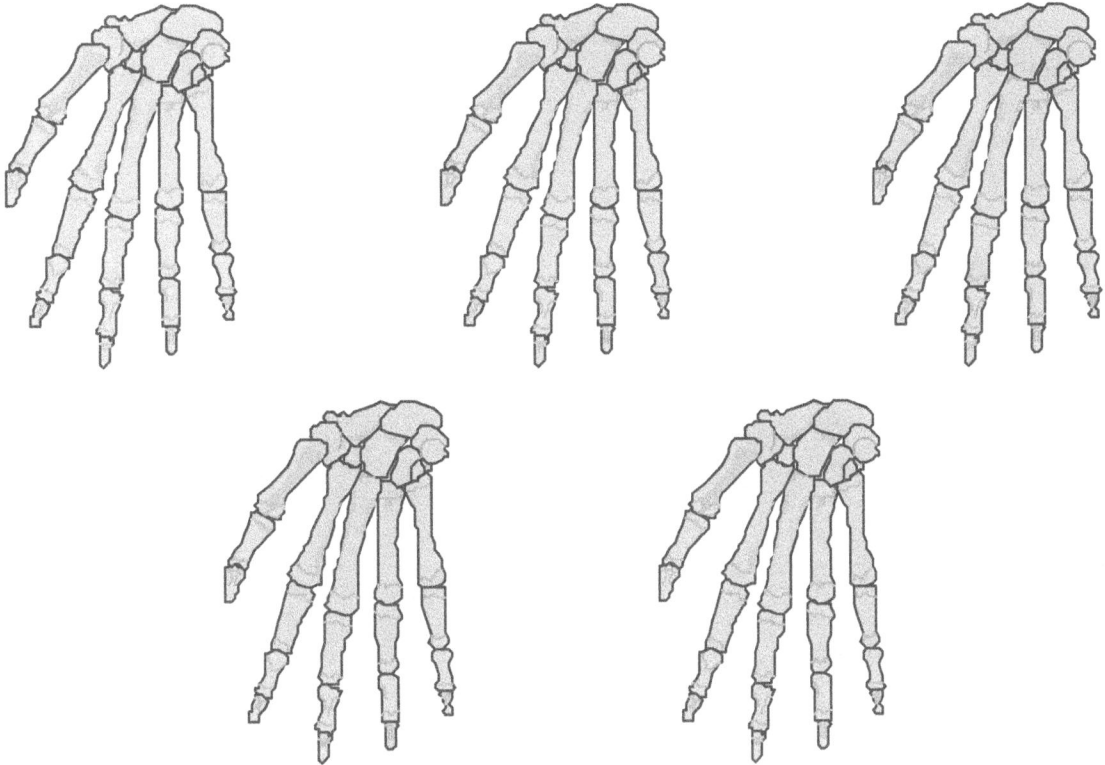

Skeletal structure of hands

Muscles on the posterior surface of the hand:

1. Dorsal Interossei

Draw the muscles on the diagram below:

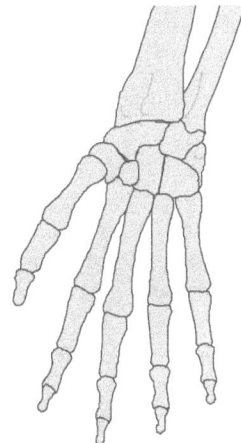

Fill in the blanks in the charts below:

Flexors of the Wrist	Origins	Insertions	Actions	Innervation of the Muscle	Nerve Root Level
Palmaris Longus					
Flexor Carpi Radialis					
Flexor Carpi Ulnaris					

Extensors of the Wrist	Origins	Insertions	Actions	Innervation of the Muscle	Nerve Root Level
Extensor Carpi Radialis Brevis					
Extensor Carpi Radialis Longus					
Extensor Carpi Ulnaris					

Radial Deviators	Origins	Insertions	Actions	Innervation of the Muscle	Nerve Root Level
Flexor Carpi Radialis					
Extensor Carpi Radialis Longus					

Ulnar Deviators	Origins	Insertions	Actions	Innervation of the Muscle	Nerve Root Level
Extensor Carpi Ulnaris					
Flexor Carpi Ulnaris					

Finger Flexors	Origins	Insertions	Actions	Innervation of the Muscle	Nerve Root Level
Flexor Pollicis Brevis					
Flexor Pollicis Longus					
Lumbricals					
Dorsal Interossei					
Palmar Interossei					
Flexor Digitorum Profundus					
Flexor Digitorum Superficialis					

Finger Extensors	Origins	Insertions	Actions	Innervation of the Muscle	Nerve Root Level
Extensor Pollicis Brevis					
Extensor Pollicis Longus					
Extensor Digitorum					
Extensor Digiti Minimi					
Extensor Indicis					
Lumbricals					
Palmar Interossei					
Dorsal Interossei					

Finger Abductors	Origins	Insertions	Actions	Innervation of the Muscle	Nerve Root Level
Abductor Pollicis Longus					
Abductor Pollicis Brevis					
Dorsal Interossei					
Abductor Digiti Minimi					

Finger Adductors	Origins	Insertions	Actions	Innervation of the Muscle	Nerve Root Level
Adductor Pollicis					
Palmar Interossei					

Opposition Muscles	Origins	Insertions	Actions	Innervation of the Muscle	Nerve Root Level
Opponens Pollicis					
Opponens Digiti Minimi					

On the diagrams below, color the area(s) that are innervated by the nerves mentioned above:

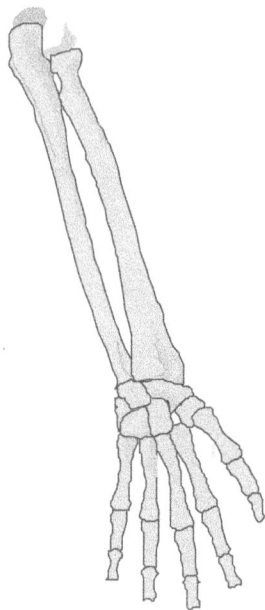

Posterior view

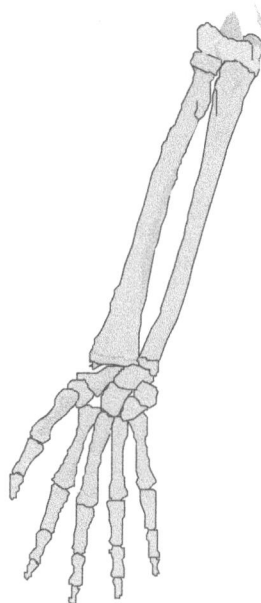

Anterior view

CONNECTIVE TISSUE

The main ligaments of the wrist and hand include:

1. Radial Collateral

2. Volar Radiocarpal

3. Ulnocarpal Ligamentous Complex

4. Dorsal Radiocarpal

5. Volar Intercarpal

6. Dorsal Intercarpal

7. Deep Transverse metacarpal

8. Phalangeal Collateral

9. Phalangeal Cruciate

10. Palmar Plates

Fill in the blanks in the chart below:

Ligament	Stabilizes What Joint	Location	Function	Clinical Presentation When Laxity Is Present
Radial Collateral				
Volar Radiocarpal				
Ulnocarpal Ligamentous Complex				
Dorsal Radiocarpal				
Volar Intercarpal				
Dorsal Intercarpal				
Deep Transverse Metacarpal				
Phalangeal Collateral				
Phalangeal Cruciate				
Palmar Plates				

Draw the ligaments on the skeletons below:

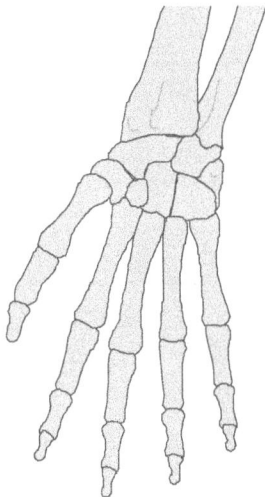

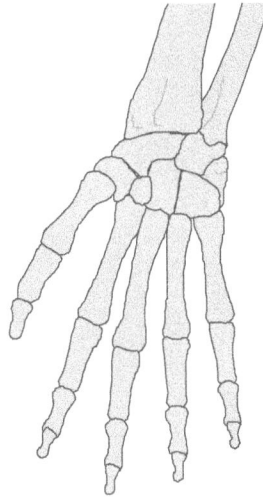

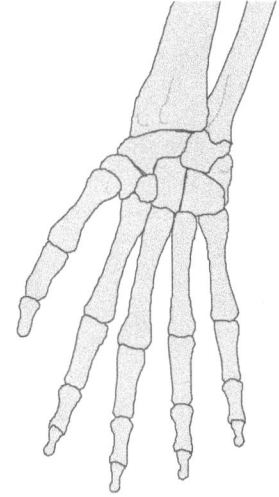

What is the purpose of the following?

1. Extensor Retinaculum

2. Flexor Retinaculum

3. Palmar Aponeurosis

ARTHROKINEMATICS ───────────────────────────────

What is the closed pack position of the wrist?

What is the loose pack position of the wrist?

Fill in the correct range of motion measurements:

Wrist Flexion _____

Wrist Extension _____

Radial Deviation _____

Ulnar Deviation _____

Metacarpophalangeal (MCP) Flexion _____

Metacarpophalangeal (MCP) Extension _____

Proximal Interphalangeal (PIP) Flexion _____

Distal Interphalangeal (DIP) Flexion _____

Distal Interphalangeal (DIP) Extension _____

Proximal Interphalangeal (PIP) Extension _____

Define the anatomical snuff box. What structures are located within it? What tendons constitute its boundaries?

Describe the following arches of the hand:

Carpal Transverse:

Metatarsal Transverse:

Longitudinal:

Describe the following grips:

Hook:

Cylinder:

Spherical:

Power:

Describe the following prehensions:

Tip to tip: Chuck (three-fingered):

Lateral key:

COMMON TREATED DIAGNOSIS OF THE WRIST AND HAND JOINT ————

1. Colle's Fractures

2. Carpal Tunnel Syndrome

3. Boutonniere Deformity

4. Scaphoid Fractures

5. Ulnar Nerve Entrapment

6. Peripheral Nerve Injuries

7. DeQuervain's Tenosynovitis

8. Dupuytren's Contracture

9. Ligamentous Injuries

10. Fractures

11. Total Joint Replacement

12. Arthritis

13. Game Keeper's Thumb

Using the *Guide* and your orthopedic textbook, fill in the chart below for each of the pathologies:

Pathology	Tissues Affected	Pathophysiology	Clinical Presentations	Preferred Practice Pattern
Colle's Fractures				
Carpal Tunnel Syndrome				
Boutonniere Deformity				
Scaphoid Fractures				
Ulnar Nerve Entrapment				
Peripheral Nerve Injuries				
DeQuervain's Tenosynovitis				
Dupuytren's Contracture				
Ligamentous Injuries				
Fractures				
Total Joint Replacement				
Arthritis				
Game Keeper's Thumb				

Common Orthopedic Tests of the Wrist and Hand

1. Murphy's Sign
2. Finkelstein's Test
3. Tinel's Sign

4. Phalen's Test
5. Reverse Phalen's Test

ORTHOPEDIC TESTS AND MEASURES —————————————————————————

Special Tests	How Is the Test Performed	A Positive Sign Looks Like	Anatomical Structure Being Tested
Murphy's Sign			
Finkelstein's Test			
Tinel's Sign			
Phalen's Test			
Reverse Phalen's Test			

TESTS AND MEASURES —————————————————————————————

Using the *Guide*, determine the appropriate tests and measures for each of the following diagnoses:

Pathology	Tests and Measures	What Is the Test and Measure Testing	Possible Abnormal Findings
Colle's Fractures			
Carpal Tunnel Syndrome			
Boutonniere Deformity			
Scaphoid Fractures			
Ulnar Nerve Entrapment			
Peripheral Nerve Injuries			
DeQuervain's Tenosynovitis			
Dupuytren's Contracture			
Ligamentous Injuries			
Fractures			
Total Joint Replacement			
Arthritis			
Game Keeper's Thumb			

INTERVENTIONS

Pathology	Interventions	Indication for Interventions	Goals of Intervention	Contraindications for Interventions	Settings for Interventions
Example	Ultrasound	Increase in pain, edema, and an increase in inflammatory response.	To decrease pain, decrease inflammatory response, and increase circulation to facilitate healing.	Pacemakers, cancer, plastic implants, pregnancy, joint cement, decreased sensation, and mentation.	Will use a pulsed ultrasound 1 MHz at 2.0 w/cm^2 at 100 percent duty cycle × 10 minutes. Phonophoresis may be beneficial as well.
Colle's Fractures					
Carpal Tunnel Syndrome					
Boutonniere Deformity					
Scaphoid Fractures					
Ulnar Nerve Entrapment					
Peripheral Nerve Injuries					
DeQuervain's Tenosynovitis					
Dupuytren's Contracture					
Ligamentous Injuries					
Fractures					
Total Joint Replacement					
Arthritis					
Game Keeper's Thumb					

Chapter 7

Hip

ANATOMY ————————————————————————————————————

Skeletal System:

1. Femur

2. Innominate
   a. The innominate is made up of the ilium, ischium, and pubis.

b. The acetabulum is made up of the ilium, ischium, and pubis.

Label the bones above on the diagram below:

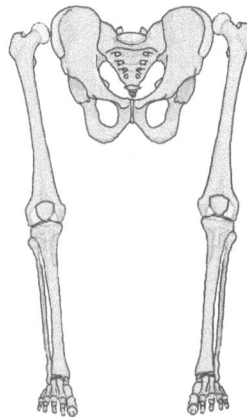

Hip and leg skeleton

Label the following bony landmarks on the diagram above:

Anterior Superior Iliac Spine

Anterior Inferior Iliac Spine

Posterior Superior Iliac Spine

Posterior Inferior Iliac Spine

Head of Femur

Greater Trochanter

Lesser Trochanter

Linea Aspera

Ischial Tuberosity

Pubic Symphysis

Medial Epicondyles and Condyles

Tibial Tuberosity

Sciatic Notch

Lateral Epicondyles and Condyles

Adductor Tubercle

Iliac Crest

Muscular System:

Muscles anterior of the hip:

1. Rectus Femoris

2. Vastus Medialis

3. Vastus Lateralis

4. Sartorius

5. Gracilis

6. Adductor Magnus

7. Adductor Longus

Draw the above muscles on the diagrams below:

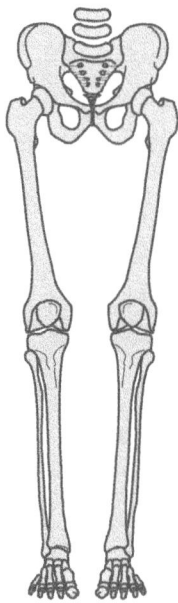

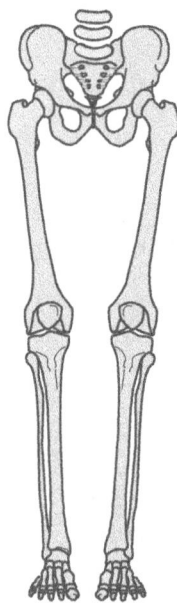

Anterior view

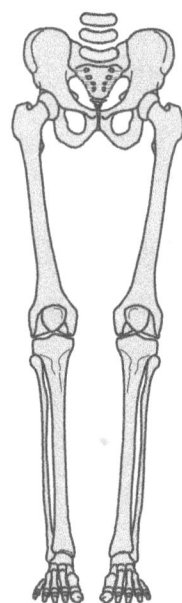

Muscles posterior of the hip:

1. Gluteus Maximus

2. Gluteus Medius

3. Gluteus Minimus

4. Biceps Femoris

5. Semitendinosus

6. Semimembranosus

7. Adductor Magnus

8. Piriformis

9. Gemellus Superior

10. Gemellus Inferior

11. Quadratus Femoris

12. Obturator Internus

13. Obturator Externus

Draw the above muscles on the diagrams below:

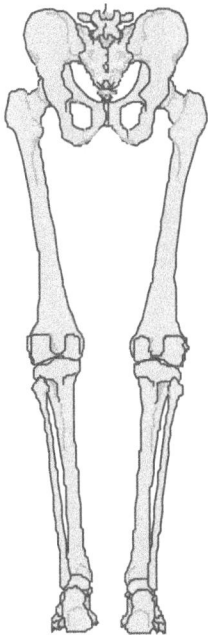

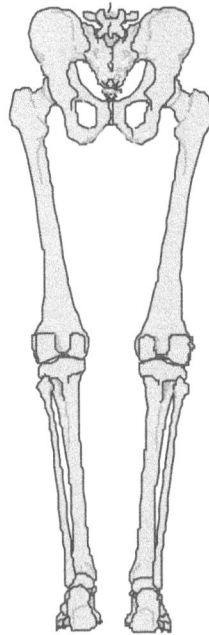

Posterior view

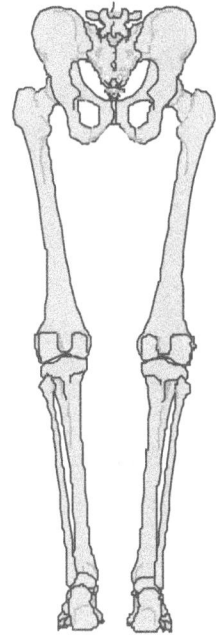

Muscles medial of the hip:

1. Adductor Longus

2. Adductor Brevis

3. Adductor Magnus

4. Gracilis

5. Vastus Medius Obliques

6. Semimembranosus

7. Pectineus

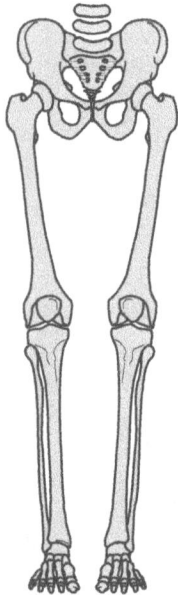 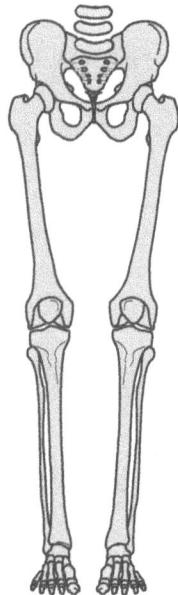 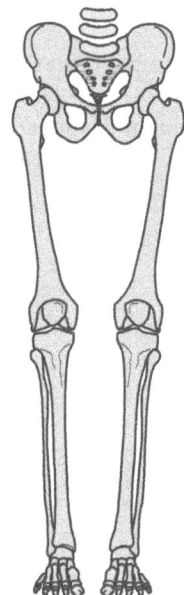

Muscles lateral of the hip:

1. Tensor Fascia Latae

2. Gluteus Medius

3. Gluteus Minimus

4. Biceps Femoris

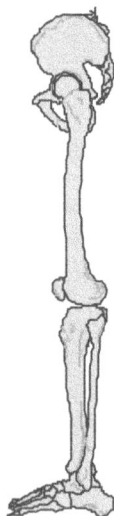 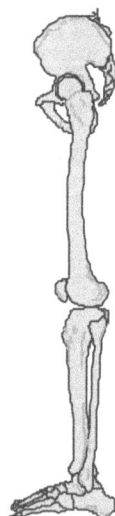 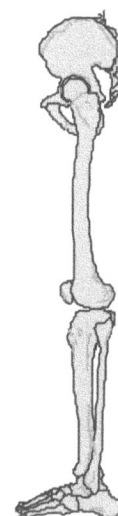

Lateral view

Fill in the blanks in the charts below:

Flexors of the Hip	Origin	Insertion	Innervation of the Muscle	Nerve Root Level
Iliopsoas				
Rectus Femoris				
Pectineus				
Sartorius				
Tensor Fascia Latae				

Extensors of the Hip	Origin	Insertion	Innervation of the Muscle	Nerve Root Level
Gluteus Maximus				
Hamstrings				
Adductor Magnus				

Internal Rotators of the Hip	Origin	Insertion	Innervation of the Muscle	Nerve Root Level
Adductor Magnus				
Adductor Longus				
Adductor Brevis				
Pectineus				
Gracilis				
Gluteus Medius				
Gluteus Minimus				

External Rotators of the Hip	Origin	Insertion	Innervation of the Muscle	Nerve Root Level
Piriformis				
Gemellus Inferior				
Gemellus Superior				
Obturator Internus				
Obturator Externus				
Quadratus Femoris				
Gluteus Medius (Posterior Fibers)				

Abductors of the Hip	Origin	Insertion	Innervation of the Muscle	Nerve Root Level
Gluteus Medius				
Gluteus Minimus				
Gluteus Maximus				
Tensor Fascia Latae				
Sartorius				

Adductors of the Hip	Origin	Insertion	Innervation of the Muscle	Nerve Root Level
Adductor Magnus				
Adductor Longus				
Adductor Brevis				
Pectineus				
Gracilis				

On the diagrams below, color the area(s) that are innervated by the nerves mentioned in the charts previous:

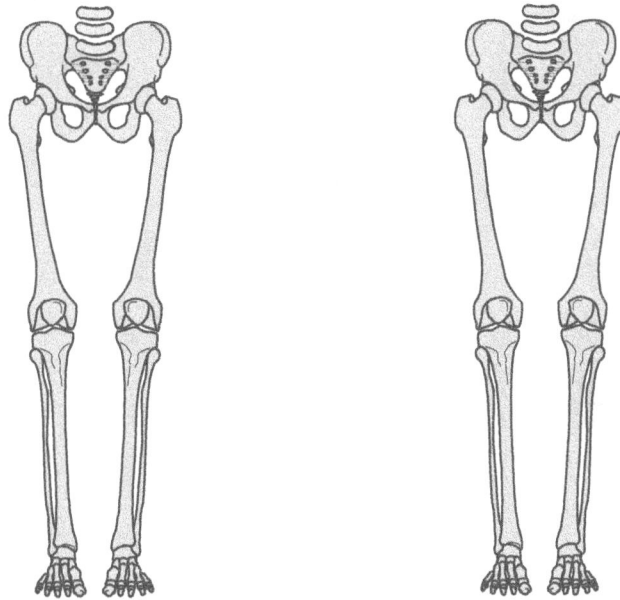

CONNECTIVE TISSUE

The main ligaments of the hip and pelvis include:

1. Iliofemoral

2. Ischiofemoral

3. Pubofemoral

4. Round

5. Sacrotuberous

6. Sacrospinous

7. Iliolumbar

8. Sacroiliac

Fill in the blanks in the chart below:

Ligaments	Location	Function	Clinical Presentation When Laxity Is Present
Iliofemoral			
Ischiofemoral			
Pubofemoral			
Round			

Ligaments	Location	Function	Clinical Presentation When Laxity Is Present
Sacrotuberous			
Sacrospinous			
Iliolumbar			
Sacroiliac			

BURSA

The Trochanteric bursa is found at the insertion of the gluteus maximus muscle.

ARTHROKINEMATICS

What is the closed pack position of the hip?

What is the loose pack position of the hip?

Fill in the correct range of motion measurements:

Hip Flexion _____

Hip Extension _____

Hip Abduction _____

Hip Adduction _____

Hip Internal Rotation _____

Hip External Rotation _____

If you are standing doing a squat, and you are focusing on your hip, when squatting, are you moving convex on concave or concave on convex? What direction is the roll? The glide?

Differentiate between coxa valgus and varum:

Define the following:

Anteversion:

Retroversion:

COMMONLY TREATED DIAGNOSES OF THE HIP AND PELVIS JOINT ———

1. Bursitis

2. Tendonitis

3. Muscle Strain

4. Femoral Fractures

5. Acetabulum Fractures

6. Total Hip Replacement

7. Arthritis

8. Hip Dislocations

9. Piriformis Syndrome

10. Myositis Ossificans

11. Sacroiliac Dysfunctions

12. Pelvic Dysfunctions

Using the *Guide* and your orthopedic textbook, fill in the chart below for each pathology:

Pathology	Tissues Affected	Pathophysiology	Clinical Presentations	Preferred Practice Pattern
Bursitis				
Tendonitis				
Muscle Strain				
Femoral Fractures				
Acetabulum Fractures				
Total Hip Replacement				
Arthritis				
Hip Dislocations				
Piriformis Syndrome				
Myositis Ossificans				
Sacroiliac Dysfunctions				
Pelvic Dysfunctions				

ORTHOPEDIC TESTS OF THE HIP

1. Scour's Test
2. Faber's Test (Patrick's Test, Figure 4 Test)
3. Ober's Test
4. Thomas Test
5. Stork Test (Gillette's Test)

6. Craig's Test
7. Straight Leg Test
8. Trendelenburg's Test
9. Ortolani

Orthopedic Special Test	How Is the Test Performed	A Positive Sign Looks Like	Anatomical Structure Being Tested
Scour's Test			
Faber's Test			
Ober's Test			

Orthopedic Special Test	How Is the Test Performed	A Positive Sign Looks Like	Anatomical Structure Being Tested
Thomas Test			
Stork Test (Gillett's Test)			
Craig's Test			
Straight Leg Test			

Orthopedic Special Test	How Is the Test Performed	A Positive Sign Looks Like	Anatomical Structure Being Tested
Trendelenburg's Test			
Ortolani			

TESTS AND MEASURES PERFORMED ON THE HIP AND PELVIS

Pathology	Tests and Measures	What Is the Test and Measure Testing?	Possible Abnormal Findings
Bursitis			
Tendonitis			
Muscle Strain			
Femoral Fractures			
Acetabulum Fractures			

Pathology	Tests and Measures	What Is the Test and Measure Testing?	Possible Abnormal Findings
Total Hip Replacement			
Arthritis			
Hip Dislocations			
Piriformis Syndrome			
Myositis Ossificans			
Sacroiliac Dysfunctions			
Pelvic Dysfunctions			

INTERVENTIONS —————————————————————————————

Pathology	Intervention	Indication for Intervention	Goals for the Intervention	Contraindications of the Intervention	Settings for Intervention
Example	Ultrasound	Increase in pain, edema, and an increase in inflammatory response.	To decrease pain, decrease inflammatory response, and increase circulation to facilitate healing.	Pacemakers, cancer, plastic implants, pregnancy, joint cement, decreased sensation and mentation.	Will use a pulsed ultrasound 1 MHz at 2.0 w/cm^2 at 100 percent duty cycle × 10 minutes. Phonophoresis may be beneficial as well.
Bursitis					
Muscle Strain					
Tendonitis					

Pathology	Intervention	Indication for Intervention	Goals for the Intervention	Contraindications of the Intervention	Settings for Intervention
Femoral Fractures					
Acetabulum Fractures					

Pathology	Intervention	Indication for Intervention	Goals for the Intervention	Contraindications of the Intervention	Settings for Intervention
Total Hip Replacement					
Arthritis					
Hip Dislocations					

Pathology	Intervention	Indication for Intervention	Goals for the Intervention	Contraindications of the Intervention	Settings for Intervention
Piriformis Syndrome					
Myositis Ossificans					
Sacroiliac Dysfunctions					
Pelvic Dysfunctions					

Chapter 8

KNEE

ANATOMY

Skeletal System:

1. Femur

2. Patella

3. Tibia

Label the bones above on the diagram below:

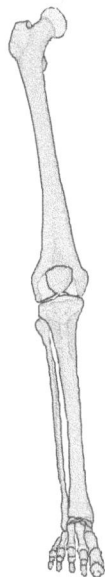

Skeletal structure of right leg

Label the following bony landmarks on the diagram above:

Patellar Base

Tibial Tuberosity

Femoral Medial Condyle

Femoral Medial Epicondyle

Tibial Lateral Condyle

Patella Apex

Fibular Head

Femoral Lateral Condyle

Femoral Lateral Epicondyle

Tibial Medial Condyle

Muscular System:

Muscles anterior of the knee:

1. Rectus Femoris
2. Vastus Medialis
3. Vastus Lateralis
4. Sartorius

5. Gracilis
6. Adductor Magnus
7. Adductor Longus

Draw the above muscles on the diagrams below:

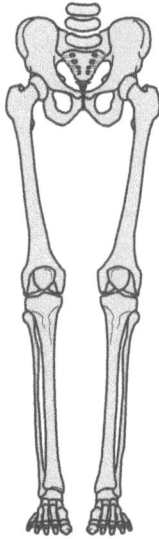

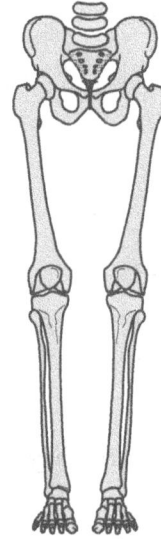

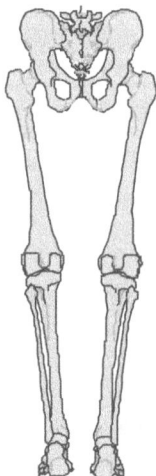

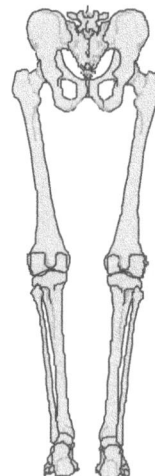

Anterior view

Muscles posterior of the knee:

1. Biceps Femoris
2. Semitendinosus

3. Semimembranosus
4. Adductor Magnus

Draw the above muscles on the diagrams below:

Posterior view

Draw the muscles below on the diagrams below:

Muscles medial of the knee:

  1. Gracilis

  2. Vastus Medius Obliques

  3. Semimembranosus

  4. Semitendinosus

Muscles lateral of the knee:

  1. Tensor Fascia Latae

  2. Gluteus Medius

  3. Gluteus Minimus

  4. Biceps Femori

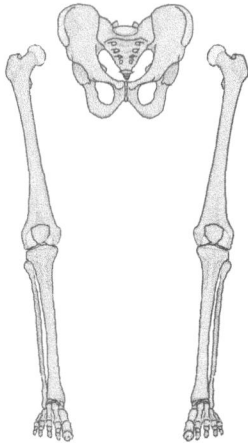

Anterior view

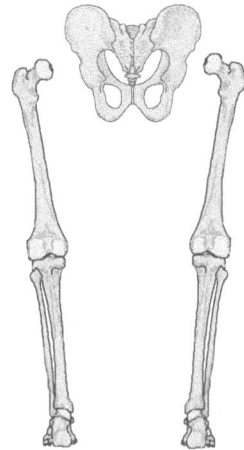

Posterior view

Fill in the blanks in the charts below:

Flexors of the Knee	Origin	Insertion	Innervation of the Muscle	Nerve Root Level
Biceps Femoris				
Semitendinosus				
Semimembranosus				
Sartorius				
Tensor Fascia Latae				
Gastrocnemius				

Extensors of the Knee	Origin	Insertion	Innervation of the Muscle	Nerve Root Level
Rectus Femoris				
Vastus Lateralis				
Vastus Medialis				
Vastus Intermedialis				

On the diagrams below, color the area(s) that are innervated by the nerves mentioned above:

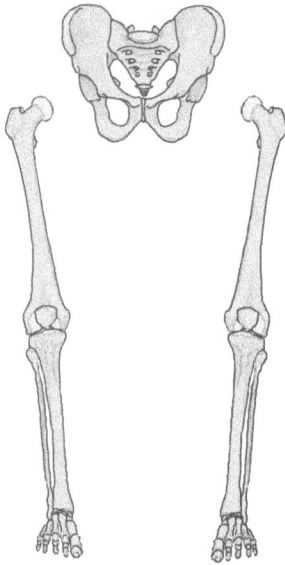

Anterior view

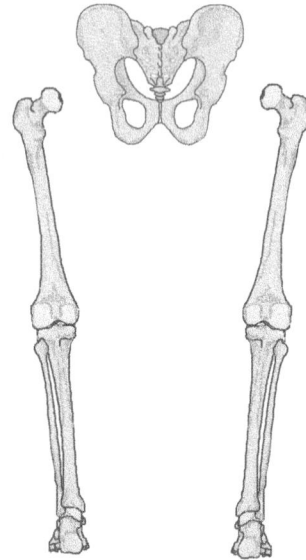

Posterior view

CONNECTIVE TISSUE ———————————————————————————

The main ligaments of the knee include:

1. Anterior Cruciate Ligament

2. Posterior Cruciate Ligament

3. Medial Collateral Ligament

4. Lateral Collateral Ligament

5. Transverse (Meniscal) Ligament

6. Coronary Ligament

Fill in the blanks in the charts below:

Ligaments	Stabilizes What Joint	Location	Function	Clinical Presentation When Laxity Is Present
Anterior Cruciate Ligament				
Posterior Cruciate Ligament				

Ligaments	Stabilizes What Joint	Location	Function	Clinical Presentation When Laxity Is Present
Medial Collateral Ligament				
Lateral Collateral Ligament				
Transverse (Meniscal) Ligament				
Coronary Ligament				

BURSA

There are numerous bursa found around the knee. Place on the diagrams below the positions of the following bursa:

Subcutaneous Prepatellar Bursa   Deep Infrapatellar Bursa

Subcutaneous Infrapatellar Bursa   Pes Anserine Bursa

Suprapatellar Bursa   Semimembranosus Bursa

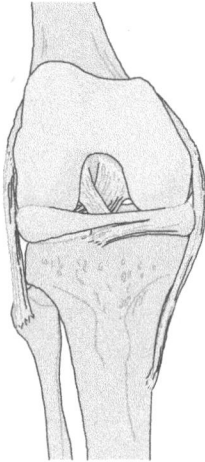

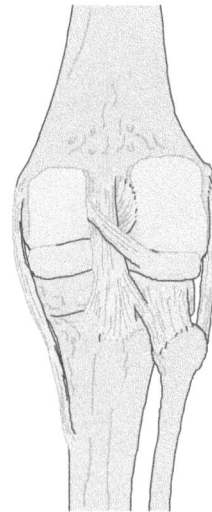

ARTHROKINEMATICS

What is the closed pack position of the knee?

What is the loose pack position of the knee?

Fill in the correct range of motion measurements:

Knee Flexion _____

Knee Extension _____

Tibial Internal Rotation _____

Tibial External Rotation _____

If you are on your hands and knees (quadruped position) and rocking back and forth, and you are focusing on your knees, are you moving convex on concave or concave on convex? What direction is the roll? The glide?

Differentiate between genu valgus and varus:

Explain the screw home mechanism. How does this differ in the weight bearing and nonweight bearing positions?

COMMON TREATED DIAGNOSIS OF THE KNEE ————————————————

1. Bursitis

2. Tendonitis

3. Muscle Strain

4. Fractures

5. Total Knee Replacement

6. Arthritis

7. Patellar Dislocations

8. Osgood Schlatter's Disease

9. Meniscal Injuries

10. Patello-femoral Dysfunction

11. Baker's Cyst

12. Ligament Injuries

Using the *Guide* and your orthopedic textbook, fill in the chart below for each pathology:

Pathology	Tissues Affected	Pathophysiology	Clinical Presentations	Preferred Practice Pattern
Bursitis				
Tendonitis				

Pathology	Tissues Affected	Pathophysiology	Clinical Presentations	Preferred Practice Pattern
Muscle Strain				
Fractures				
Total Knee Replacement				
Arthritis				
Osgood Schlatter's Disease				

Pathology	Tissues Affected	Pathophysiology	Clinical Presentations	Preferred Practice Pattern
Patellar Dislocations				
Meniscal Injuries				
Patello-femoral Dysfunction				
Baker's Cyst				
Ligament Injuries				

COMMON ORTHOPEDIC TESTS OF THE KNEE ————————————————————

1. Valgus Stress Test
2. Varus Stress Test
3. Anterior Drawer Test
4. Posterior Drawer Test
5. Posterior Sag Test
6. Lachman's Test

7. McMurray's Test
8. Apley Grind Test
9. Apley Distraction Test
10. Bounce Home (Spring Test)
11. Patellar Apprehension Test
12. Clarke's Sign

Orthopedic Tests	How the Test Is Performed	A Positive Sign Looks Like:	Anatomical Structure Being Tested
Valgus Stress Test			
Varus Stress Test			
Anterior Drawer Test			
Posterior Drawer Test			

Orthopedic Tests	How the Test Is Performed	A Positive Sign Looks Like:	Anatomical Structure Being Tested
Posterior Sag Test			
Lachman's Test			
McMurray's Test			
Apley Grind Test			
Apley Distraction Test			

Orthopedic Tests	How the Test Is Performed	A Positive Sign Looks Like:	Anatomical Structure Being Tested
Bounce Home (Spring Test)			
Patellar Apprehension Test			
Clarke's Sign			

OTHER TESTS AND MEASURES OF THE KNEE

Pathology	Tests and Measures	What Is the Test and Measure Testing?	Possible Abnormal Findings
Bursitis			
Tendonitis			

Pathology	Tests and Measures	What Is the Test and Measure Testing?	Possible Abnormal Findings
Muscle Strain			
Fractures			
Total Knee Replacement			
Arthritis			
Patellar Dislocations			

Pathology	Tests and Measures	What Is the Test and Measure Testing?	Possible Abnormal Findings
Osgood Schlatter's Disease			
Meniscal Injuries			
Patello-femoral Dysfunction			
Baker's Cyst			
Ligament Injuries			

INTERVENTIONS

Pathology	Intervention	Indication for Intervention	Goals for the Intervention	Contraindications of the Intervention	Settings for Intervention
	Ultrasound	Increase in pain, edema, and an increase in inflammatory response.	To decrease pain, decrease inflammatory response, and increase circulation to facilitate healing.	Pacemakers, cancer, plastic implants, pregnancy, joint cement, and decreased sensation and mentation.	Will use a pulsed ultrasound 1 MHz at 2.0 w/cm^2 at 100% duty cycle × 10 minutes. Phonophoresis may be beneficial as well.
Bursitis					
Tendonitis					
Muscle Strain					
Pathology					

Pathology	Intervention	Indication for Intervention	Goals for the Intervention	Contraindications of the Intervention	Settings for Intervention
Fractures					
Total Knee Replacement					
Arthritis					
Patellar Dislocations					
Osgood Schlatter's Disease					

Pathology	Intervention	Indication for Intervention	Goals for the Intervention	Contraindications of the Intervention	Settings for Intervention
Meniscal Injuries					
Patello-femoral Dysfunction					
Baker's Cyst					
Ligament Injuries					

Chapter 9

FOOT AND ANKLE

ANATOMY

Skeletal System:

1. Tibia

2. Fibula

3. Calcaneous

4. Talus

5. Navicular

6. Cuboid

7. Cuniform I

8. Cuniform II

9. Cuniform III

10. Metatarsals

11. Phalanges

Label the listed bones on the diagram below:

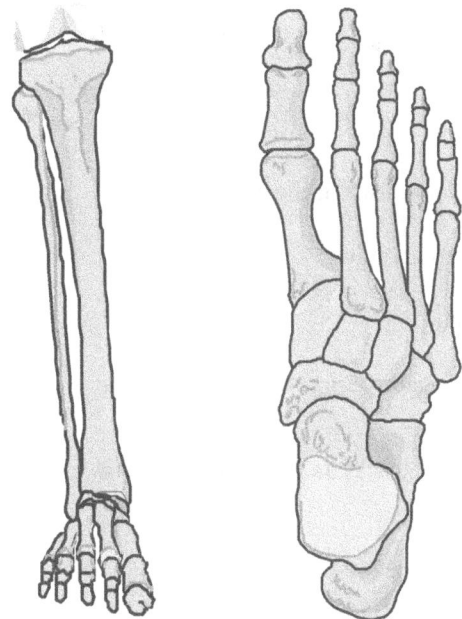

Skeletal leg and foot

Label the following bony landmarks on the diagrams above:

Lateral Malleolus	Sustenaculum Tali
Medial Malleolus	Metatarsal Head
Navicular Tuberosity	Metatarsal Base
Phalangeal Head	Phalangeal Base
Phalangeal Shaft	Metatarsal Shaft

Muscular System:

Muscles anterior of the ankle:

1. Anterior Tibialis

2. Extensor Digitorum

3. Extensor Hallucis Longus

Draw the above muscles on the diagrams below:

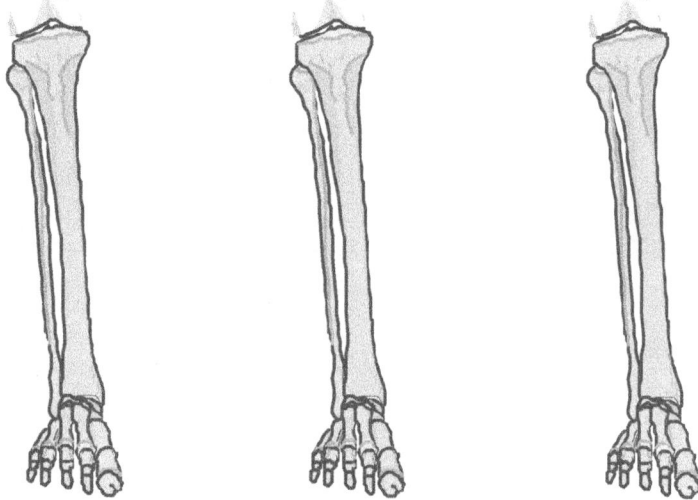

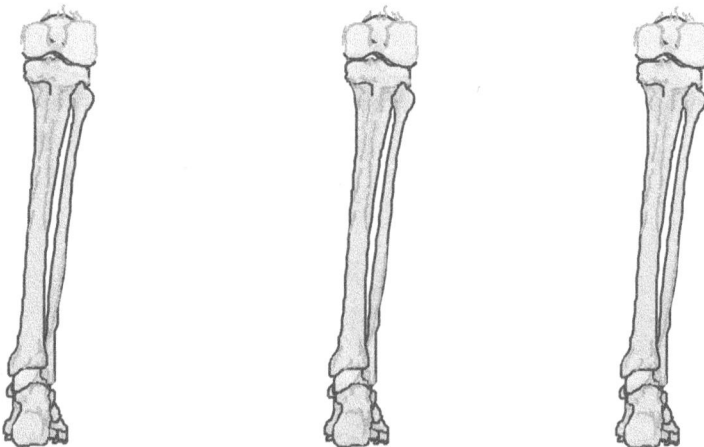

Anterior view

Muscles posterior of the ankle:

1. Gastrocnemius

2. Soleus

3. Tibialis Posterior

4. Plantaris

5. Flexor Hallucis Longus

6. Flexor Digitorum Longus

Draw the muscles on the diagrams below:

Posterior view

Muscles medial of the lower leg:

   1. Tibialis Posterior

   2. Flexor Hallucis Longus

   3. Flexor Digitorum Longus

Muscles lateral of the lower leg:

   1. Peroneus Longus

   2. Peroneus Brevis

   3. Peroneus Tertius

Muscles of the ventral surface of the foot:

   1. Extensor Digitorum Brevis

   2. Extensor Hallucis Brevis

   3. Dorsal Interossei

   4. Plantar Interossei

   5. Lumbricals

Draw the muscles on the diagrams below:

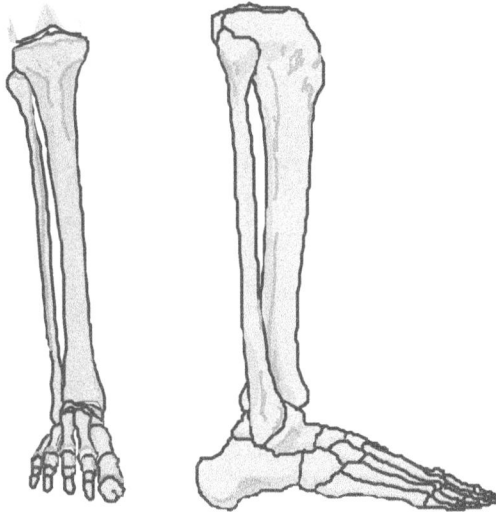

Muscles of the plantar surface of the foot:

   1. Flexor Digitorum Brevis

   2. Flexor Hallucis Brevis

   3. Flexor Digiti Minimi

   4. Abductor Hallucis

   5. Abductor Digiti Minimi

   6. Adductor Hallucis

Draw the muscles on the foot for both ventral and plantar surfaces:

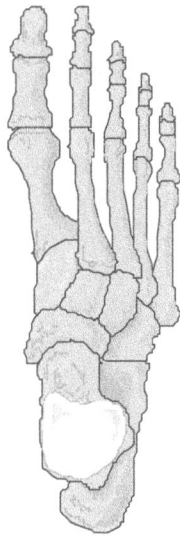

Ventral view

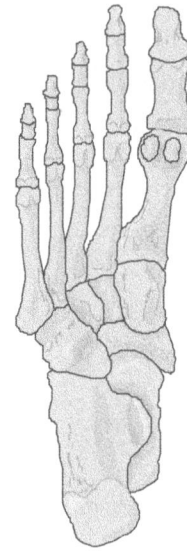

Plantar view

Fill in the blanks in the charts below:

Dorsiflexors of the Ankle	Origins	Insertions	Actions	Innervation of the Muscle	Nerve Root Level
Tibialis Anterior					
Extensor Hallucis Longus					
Extensor Digitorum Longus					
Peroneus Tertius					

Plantarflexors of the Ankle	Origins	Insertions	Actions	Innervation of the Muscle	Nerve Root Level
Gastrocnemius					
Soleus					
Tibialis Posterior					
Plantaris					
Flexor Digitorum Longus					
Flexor Hallucis Longus					

Invertors of the Ankle	Origins	Insertions	Actions	Innervation of the Muscle	Nerve Root Level
Tibialis Anterior					
Tibialis Posterior					
Flexor Digitorum Longus					
Flexor Hallucis Longus					
Extensor Hallucis Longus					

Evertors of the Ankle	Origins	Insertions	Actions	Innervation of the Muscle	Nerve Root Level
Peroneus Longus					
Peroneus Brevis					
Peroneus Tertius					

Flexors of the Toes	Origins	Insertions	Actions	Innervation of the Muscle	Nerve Root Level
Flexor Digitorum Longus					
Flexor Hallucis Longus					
Flexor Digitorum Brevis					
Flexor Hallucis Brevis					
Dorsal Interossei					
Plantar Interossei					
Flexor Digiti Minimi					
Lumbricals					

Extensors of the Toes	Origins	Insertions	Actions	Innervation of the Muscle	Nerve Root Level
Extensor Hallucis Longus					
Extensor Digitorum Longus					
Extensor Digitorum Brevis					
Lumbricals					

Abductors of the Toes	Origins	Insertions	Actions	Innervation of the Muscle	Nerve Root Level
Abductor Hallucis					
Abductor Digiti Minimi					
Dorsal Interossei					

Adductors of the Toes	Origins	Insertions	Actions	Innervation of the Muscle	Nerve Root Level
Adductor Hallucis					
Plantar Interossei					

Nervous System

On the diagrams below, color the areas that are innervated by nerves mentioned above:

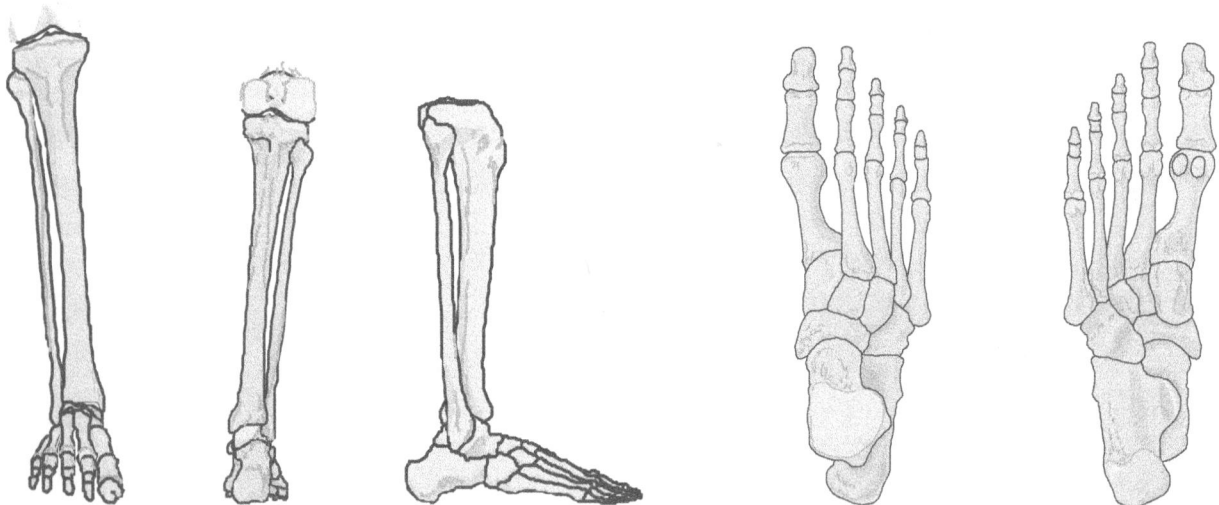

Anterior, Posterior and Lateral views of leg and foot skeleton

CONNECTIVE TISSUE

The main ligaments of the ankle include:

1. Deltoid Ligament
2. Spring Ligament
3. Anterior Tibiofibular Ligament
4. Posterior Tibiofibular Ligament
5. Anterior Talofibular Ligament
6. Posterior Talofibular Ligament
7. Interosseus Membrane
8. Bifurcated Ligament
9. Talonavicular Ligament
10. Dorsal Cuneonavicular Ligament

11. Dorsal Cuneocuboid Ligament
12. Dorsal Tarsometatarsal Ligaments
13. Dorsal Metatarsal Ligaments
14. Long Plantar Ligaments
15. Calcaneofibular Ligament
16. Plantar Metatarsal Ligaments
17. Plantar Tarsometatarsal Ligaments
18. Plantar Cuneonavicular Ligaments
19. Short Plantar Ligament

Fill in the blanks in the chart below:

Ligaments	Stabilizes What Joint	Location	Function	Clinical Presentation When Laxity Is Present
Deltoid Ligament				
Spring Ligament				

Ligaments	Stabilizes What Joint	Location	Function	Clinical Presentation When Laxity Is Present
Anterior Tibiofibular Ligament				
Posterior Tibiofibular Ligament				
Anterior Talofibular Ligament				
Posterior Talofibular Ligament				

Ligaments	Stabilizes What Joint	Location	Function	Clinical Presentation When Laxity Is Present
Interosseus Membrane				
Bifurcated Ligament				
Talonavicular Ligament				
Dorsal Cuneonavicular Ligament				

Ligaments	Stabilizes What Joint	Location	Function	Clinical Presentation When Laxity Is Present
Dorsal Cuneocuboid Ligament				
Dorsal Tarsometatarsal Ligaments				
Dorsal Metatarsal Ligaments				
Long Plantar Ligaments				

Ligaments	Stabilizes What Joint	Location	Function	Clinical Presentation When Laxity Is Present
Calcaneofibular Ligament				
Plantar Metatarsal Ligaments				
Plantar Tarsometatarsal Ligaments				
Plantar Cuneonavicular Ligaments				
Short Plantar Ligament				

Draw the ligaments of the foot below:

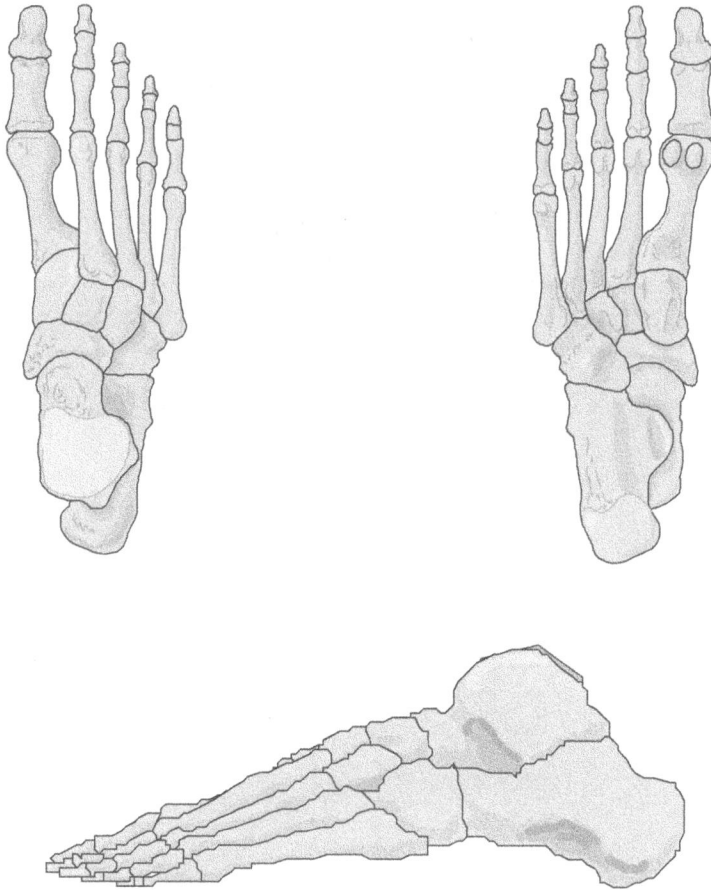

ARTHROKINEMATICS

What is the closed pack position of the talo-crural joint?

What is the loose pack position of the talo-crural joint?

Fill in the correct range of motion measurements:

Dorsiflexion   _____

Plantarflexion   _____

Inversion   _____

Eversion   _____

Toe Flexion   _____

Toe Extension   _____

If you are driving the car and press on the gas pedal, are you moving convex on concave or concave on convex at the talo-crural joint? What direction is the roll? The glide?

Describe the different rays of the foot:

1st ray:

2nd ray:

3rd ray:

4th ray:

5th ray:

Describe the following arches:

Lateral Longitudinal Arch:

Medial Longitudinal Arch:

Transverse Arch:

Differentiate between supination and pronation. How does this differ with weight bearing and nonweight bearing positions?

Define the following:

Pes Planus:

Pes Cavus:

Hindfoot Valgus:

Hindfoot Varus:

Hallux Valgus:

Claw Toes:

Hammer Toes:

Mallet Toes:

Commonly Treated Diagnoses of the Foot and Ankle

1. Achilles Tendon Tear

2. Traumatic Fractures

3. Stress Fractures

4. Tarsal Coalitions

5. Plantar Fascitis

6. Hallux Abducto Valgus (Bunions)

7. Pes Equinus

8. Tarsal Tunnel Syndrome

9. Metatarsalgia

10. Morton's Neuroma

11. Ligamentous Sprains

12. Muscle Strains

13. Shin Splints

14. Pes Cavus

15. Pes Planus

16. Arthritis

Using the *Guide* and your orthopedic textbook, fill in the chart below for each pathology:

Pathology	Tissues Affected	Pathophysiology	Clinical Presentations	Preferred Practice Pattern
Achilles Tendon Tear				
Traumatic Fractures				
Stress Fractures				
Tarsal Coalitions				
Plantar Fascitis				

Pathology	Tissues Affected	Pathophysiology	Clinical Presentations	Preferred Practice Pattern
Hallux Abducto Valgus (Bunions)				
Pes Equinus				
Tarsal Tunnel Syndrome				
Metatarsalgia				
Morton's Neuroma				
Ligamentous Sprains				

Pathology	Tissues Affected	Pathophysiology	Clinical Presentations	Preferred Practice Pattern
Muscle Strains				
Shin Splints				
Pes Cavus				
Pes Planus				
Arthritis				

Common Orthopedic Tests of the Foot and Ankle

1. Thompson's Test
2. Homan's Test
3. Kleiger's Test
4. Anterior Drawer Test

5. Tibial Torsion Test
6. Tinel's Sign
7. Talar Tilt Test

Orthopedic Tests	Procedure for Testing	Characteristics of a Positive Outcome	Anatomical Structures Being Tested
Thompson's Test			
Homan's Test			
Kleiger's Test			

Orthopedic Tests	Procedure for Testing	Characteristics of a Positive Outcome	Anatomical Structures Being Tested
Anterior Drawer Test			
Tibial Torsion Test			
Tinel's Sign			
Talar Tilt Test			

OTHER TESTS AND MEASURES PERFORMED ON THE FOOT AND ANKLE

Pathology	Tests and Measures	What Is the Test and Measure Testing?	Possible Abnormal Findings
Achilles Tendon Tear			
Traumatic Fractures			
Stress Fractures			
Tarsal Coalition			

Pathology	Tests and Measures	What Is the Test and Measure Testing?	Possible Abnormal Findings
Plantar Fascitis			
Hallux Abducto Valgus			
Pes Equinus			
Metatarsalgia			
Morton's Neuroma			

Pathology	Tests and Measures	What Is the Test and Measure Testing?	Possible Abnormal Findings
Ligamentous Sprains			
Muscle Strains			
Shin Splints			
Pes Cavus			
Pes Planus			
Arthritis			

INTERVENTIONS

Pathology	Interventions	Indications for Interventions	Goals of Intervention	Contraindications for Interventions	Settings for Intervention
Achilles Tendon Tear					
Traumatic Fractures					
Stress Fractures					
Tarsal Coalitions					
Plantar Fascitis					

Pathology	Interventions	Indications for Interventions	Goals of Intervention	Contraindications for Interventions	Settings for Intervention
Hallux Abducto Valgus (Bunions)					
Pes Equinus					
Tarsal Tunnel Syndrome					
Metatarsalgia					
Morton's Neuroma					
Ligamentous Sprains					

Pathology	Interventions	Indications for Interventions	Goals of Intervention	Contraindications for Interventions	Settings for Intervention
Muscle Strains					
Shin Splints					
Pes Cavus					
Pes Planus					
Arthritis					

Chapter 10

SPINE

ANATOMY

1. Cranium

2. Cervical Vertebra

3. Thoracic Vertebra

4. Lumbar Vertebra

5. Sacrum

6. Coccyx

Identify the parts of the spinal column on the diagram below:

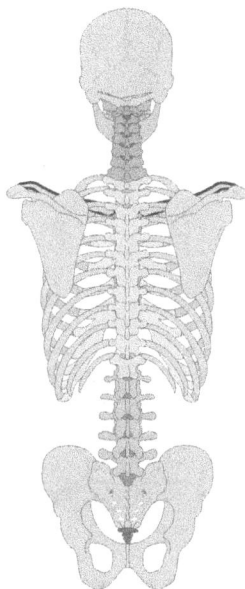

Skeletal structure of spine

Bony Landmarks

Mark the following landmarks on the diagrams below:

Cervical

1. Superior Facet

2. Inferior Facet

3. Anterior Arch

4. Posterior Arch

5. Vertebral Foramen

6. Dens (Odontoid Process)

7. Body

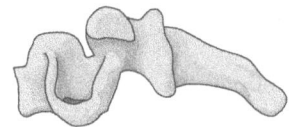

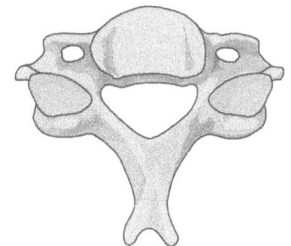

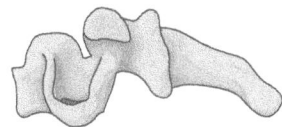

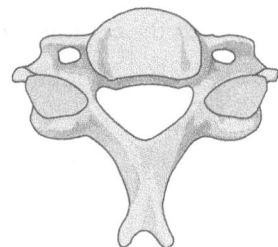

Thoracic

1. Superior Facet

2. Inferior Facet

3. Spinous Process

4. Transverse Process

5. Body

6. Lamina

7. Pedicle

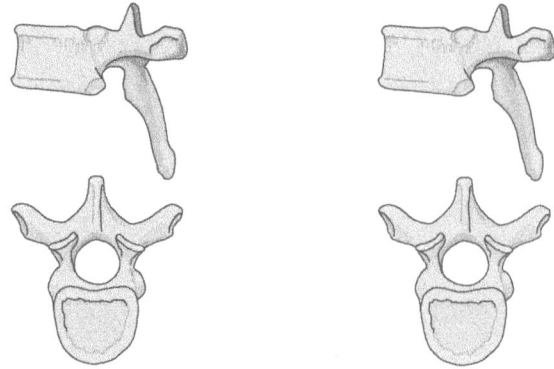

Lumbar

1. Superior Facet

2. Inferior Facet

3. Transverse Process

4. Spinous Process

5. Body

6. Pedicle

7. Lamina

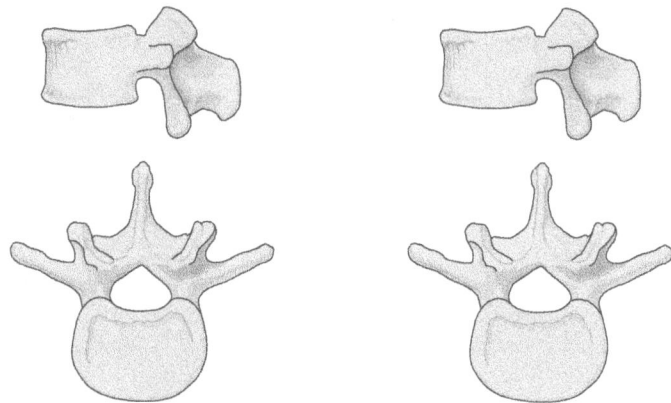

Sacrum

1. Sacral Apex

2. Sacral Promontory

3. Sacral Spinous Process

4. Sacral Base

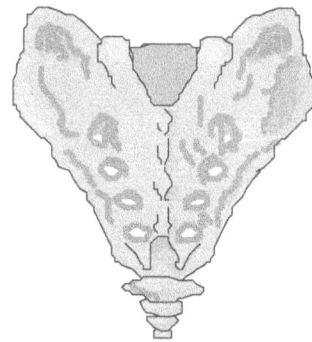

Coccyx

Compare and contrast the cervical, thoracic, and lumbar vertebra:

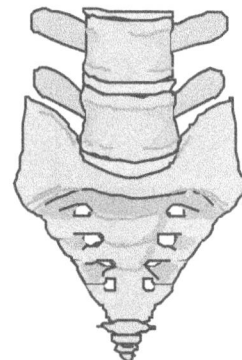

Vertebra	Number of Vertebra	Body	Superior Facets	Inferior Facets	Transverse Processes	Spinous Processes	Mobility
Cervical Vertebra							
Thoracic Vertebra							
Lumbar Vertebra							

Muscular System

Muscles anterior of the cervical spine:

1. Sternocleidomastoid

2. Scalenes

3. Longus Coli

4. Longus Cervicis

5. Rectus Capitis Anterior

Draw the above muscles on the cervical spine below:

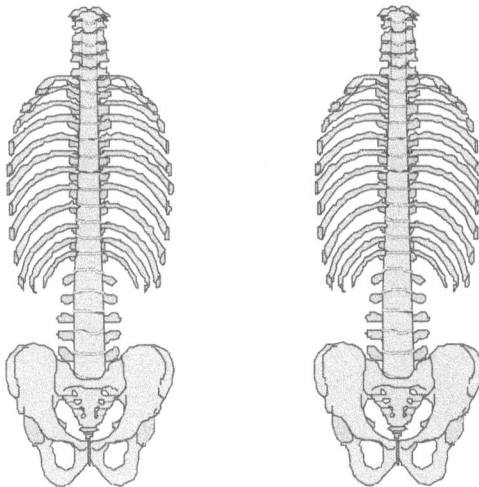

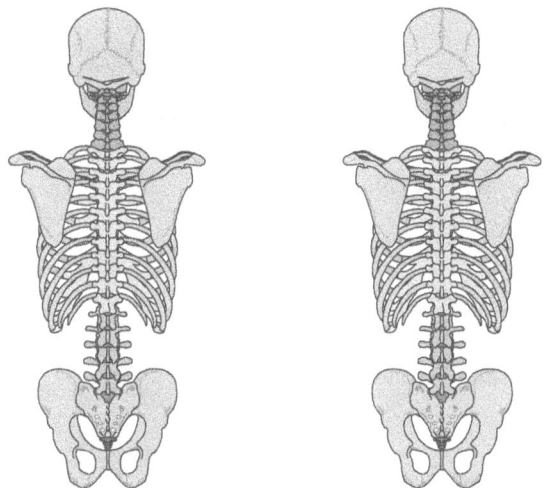

Muscles posterior of the cervical spine:

1. Rectus Capitus Posterior Major

2. Rectus Capitus Posterior Minor

3. Obliques Capitus Superior

4. Obliques Capitus Inferior

5. Splenius Capitis

6. Splenius Cervicis

7. Upper Trapezius

Draw the above muscles on the cervical spine below:

Muscles lateral of the cervical spine:

1. Rectus Capitus Lateralis

2. Rectus Capitus Anterior

3. Longus Colli

4. Longus Capitus

5. Scalenes
   a. Anterior
   b. Middle
   c. Posterior

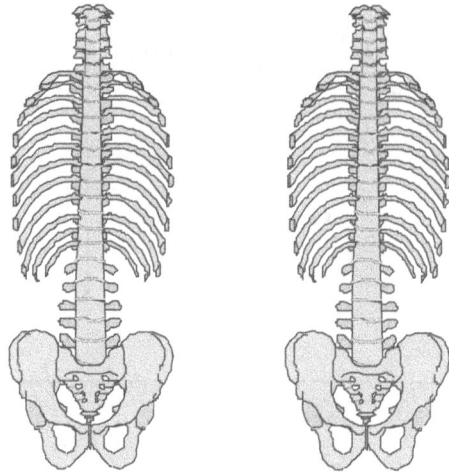

Draw the muscles on skeleton below:

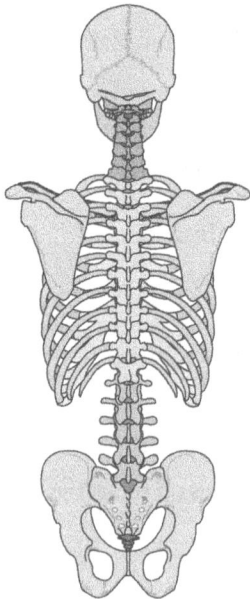

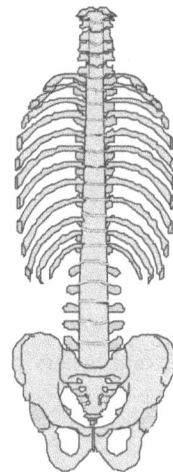

Muscles anterior of the thoracic and lumbar spine:

1. Rectus Abdominus

2. External Obliques

3. Internal Obliques

4. Transversus Abdominis

Muscles posterior of the thoracic and lumbar spine:

1. Iliocostalis

2. Longissimus

3. Spinalis

4. Interspinalis

5. Serratus Posterior Inferior

6. Serratus Posterior Superior

7. Multifidus

8. Rotatores

9. Semispinalis

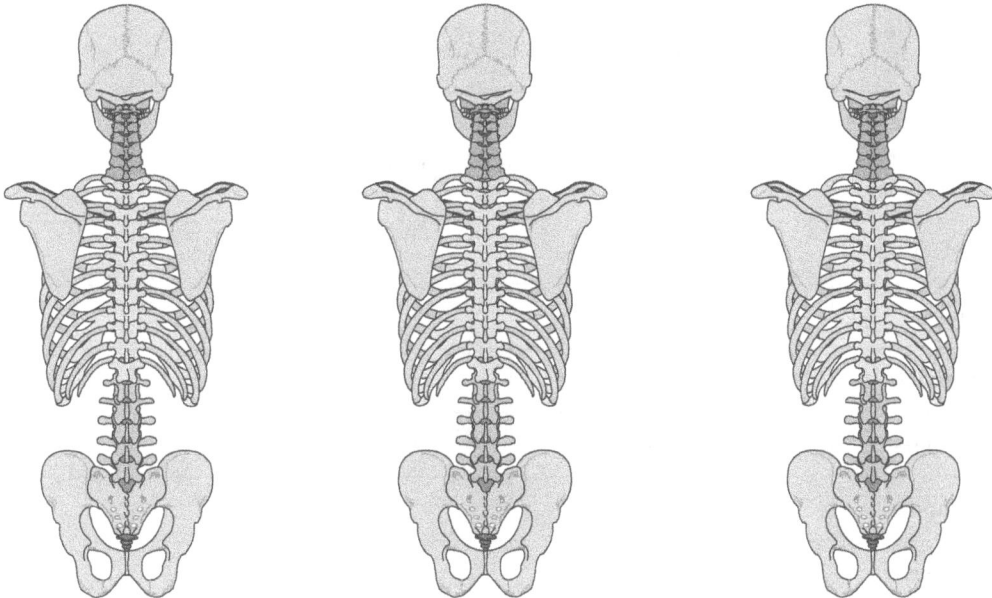

Muscles lateral of the thoracic and lumbar spine:

1. Intertransversarii

2. Quadratus Lumborum

Draw the muscles on the skeletons above:

Fill in the blanks in the charts below:

Flexors of the Cervical Spine	Origins	Insertions	Actions	Innervation of the Muscle	Nerve Root Level
Sternocleidomastoid					
Scalenes					
Longus Coli					
Longus Capitis					
Rectus Capitis Anterior					

Extensors of the Cervical Spine	Origins	Insertions	Actions	Innervation of the Muscle	Nerve Root Level
Iliocostalis Cervicis					
Longissimus Capitis					
Longissimus Cervicis					
Multifidus					
Spinalis Cervicis					
Spinalis Capitis					
Splenius Capitis					
Splenius Cervicis					
Rectus Capitis Posterior Minor					
Rectus Capitis Posterior Major					
Obliques Capitis Superior					
Obliques Capitis Inferior					

Lateral Flexors of the Cervical Spine	Origins	Insertions	Actions	Innervation of the Muscle	Nerve Root Level
Rectus Capitis Lateralis					
Scalenes					
Obliques Capitis Superior					
Iliocostalis Cervicis					

Rotators of the Cervical Spine	Origins	Insertions	Actions	Innervation of the Muscle	Nerve Root Level
Longus Coli					
Scalenes					
Obliques Capitis Inferior					
Rectus Capitis Posterior Major					

Flexors of the Thoracic/Lumbar Spine	Origins	Insertions	Actions	Innervation of the Muscle	Nerve Root Level
Internal Obliques					
External Obliques					
Rectus Abdominus					

Extensors of the Thoracic/Lumbar Spine	Origins	Insertions	Actions	Innervation of the Muscle	Nerve Root Level
Iliocostalis Lumborum					
Iliocostalis Thoracis					
Multifidus					
Rotatores					
Semispinalis Thoracis					
Spinalis Thoracis					

Lateral Flexors of the Thoracic/Lumbar Spine	Origins	Insertions	Actions	Innervation of the Muscle	Nerve Root Level
Iliocostalis Lumborum					
Iliocostalis Thoracis					
Intertransversarii					

Rotators of the Thoracic/Lumbar Spine	Origins	Insertions	Actions	Innervation of the Muscle	Nerve Root Level
Multifidus					
Rotatores					
Semispinalis Thoracis					

Connective Tissue

Using your textbook, fill in information regarding the following ligaments of the spine:

1. Anterior Longitudinal

2. Posterior Longitudinal

3. Ligamentum Flavum

4. Interspinous

5. Intertransverse

6. Supraspinous

7. Tectorial Membrane

8. Posterior Atlantoaxial

9. Ligamentum Nuchae

10. Alar

11. Iliolumbar

12. Sacrospinous

13. Sacrotuberous

14. Anterior Sacroiliac

15. Posterior Sacroiliac

Fill in the blanks in the chart below:

Ligaments	Stabilizes What Joint	Location	Function	Clinical Presentation When Laxity Is Present
Anterior Longitudinal				
Posterior Longitudinal				
Ligamentum Flavum				
Interspinous				
Intertransverse				

Ligaments	Stabilizes What Joint	Location	Function	Clinical Presentation When Laxity Is Present
Supraspinous				
Tectorial Membrane				
Posterior Atlantoaxial				
Ligamentum Nuchae				
Alar				

Ligaments	Stabilizes What Joint	Location	Function	Clinical Presentation When Laxity Is Present
Iliolumbar				
Sacrospinous				
Sacrotuberous				
Anterior Sacroiliac				
Posterior Sacroiliac				

Draw the ligaments on the skeletons below:

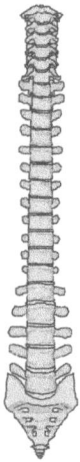

Anterior view   **Posterior view**

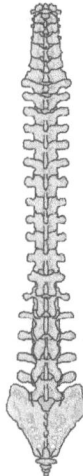

Mobility

1. Flexion and extension occurs most at the

   _____.

2. Rotation occurs most at the _____.

3. Sidebending occurs most at the

   _____.

Explain the mobility of the vertebra with the following motions:

1. Flexion

2. Extension

3. Lateral flexion (sidebending)

4. Rotation

The intervertebral disks are made up of the annulus fibrosus and the nucleus pulposus.

Draw the intervertebral disk and label the annulus fibrosus and the nucleus pulposus. Describe each part of the disk:

COMMON TREATED DIAGNOSIS OF THE SPINE ————————————————

1. Ligamentous Strain

2. Muscle Strain

3. Ruptured/Herniated Disk

4. Scoliosis

5. Kyphosis

6. Ankylosing Spondylitis

7. Spondylosis

8. Spondylolithesis

9. Compression Fractures

10. Post-Surgical Spinal Procedures

11. Thoracic Outlet Syndrome

12. Arthritis

13. Postural Dysfunctions

14. Spinal Stenosis

15. Sciatica

16. Facet Joint Dysfunctions

17. Degenerative Disk Disease

18. Nerve Compression

19. Myelopathy

20. Tumors

Using the *Guide* and your orthopedic textbook, fill in the chart below for each pathology:

Pathology	Tissues Affected	Pathophysiology	Clinical Presentations	Preferred Practice Pattern
Ligamentous Strain				
Muscle Strain				
Ruptured/ Herniated Disk				
Scoliosis				
Kyphosis				

Pathology	Tissues Affected	Pathophysiology	Clinical Presentations	Preferred Practice Pattern
Ankylosing Spondylitis				
Spondylosis				
Spondylolithesis				
Compression Fractures				
Post-Surgical Spinal Procedures				

Pathology	Tissues Affected	Pathophysiology	Clinical Presentations	Preferred Practice Pattern
Thoracic Outlet Syndrome				
Arthritis				
Postural Dysfunctions				
Spinal Stenosis				
Sciatica				

Pathology	Tissues Affected	Pathophysiology	Clinical Presentations	Preferred Practice Pattern
Facet Joint Dysfunctions				
Degenerative Disk Disease				
Nerve Compression				
Myelopathy				
Tumors				

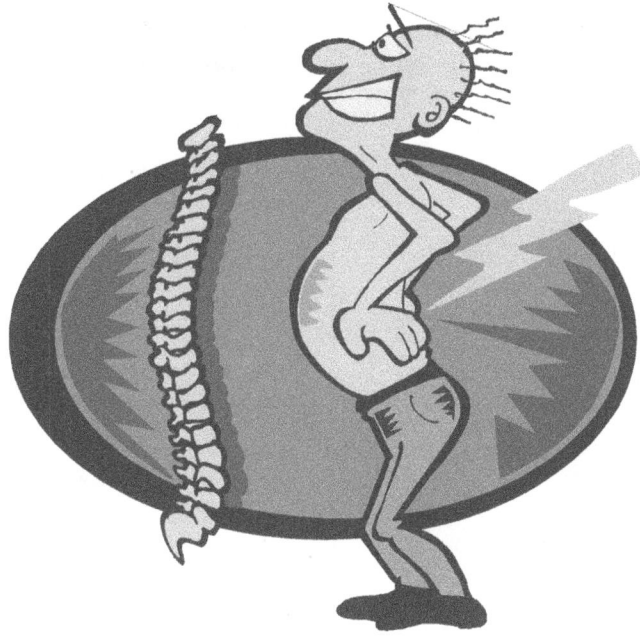

COMMON ORTHOPEDIC TESTS OF THE SPINE

1. Vertebral Artery Test

2. Foraminal Compression Test

3. Foraminal Distraction Test

4. Valsalva's Maneuver

5. Tinel's Test

6. Kernig/Brudzinski Sign

7. Anterior/Posterior Rib Compression Test

8. Lateral Rib Compression Test

9. Stoop Test

10. Hoover Test

11. Straight Leg Raise Test

12. Laseague Test

13. Slump Test

14. Spring Test

15. Trendelenburg's Test

16. Stork Gillett Test

17. Sacroiliac Joint Stress Test

18. Yeoman's Test

19. Patrick or Faber's Test

Orthopedic Tests	How the Test Is Performed	A Positive Sign Looks Like	Anatomical Structure Being Tested
Vertebral Artery Test			
Foraminal Compression Test			
Foraminal Distraction Test			
Valsalva's Maneuver			
Tinel's Test			

Orthopedic Tests	How the Test Is Performed	A Positive Sign Looks Like	Anatomical Structure Being Tested
Kernig/Brudzinski Sign			
Anterior/Posterior Rib Compression Test			
Lateral Rib Compression Test			
Stoop Test			
Hoover Test			

Orthopedic Tests	How the Test Is Performed	A Positive Sign Looks Like	Anatomical Structure Being Tested
Straight Leg Raise Test			
Laseague Test			
Slump Test			
Spring Test			
Trendelenburg's Test			

Orthopedic Tests	How the Test Is Performed	A Positive Sign Looks Like	Anatomical Structure Being Tested
Stork Gillett Test			
Sacroiliac Joint Stress Test			
Yeoman's Test			
Patrick or Faber's Test			

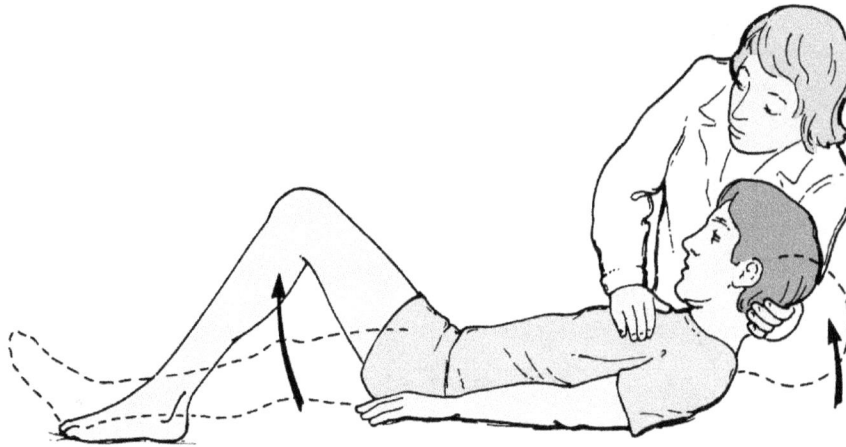

OTHER TESTS AND MEASURES OF THE SPINE ━━━━━━━━━━━━━━━━━━

Pathology	Tests and Measures	What Is the Test and Measure Testing?	Possible Abnormal Findings
Ligamentous Strain			
Muscle Strain			
Ruptured/Herniated Disk			

Pathology	Tests and Measures	What Is the Test and Measure Testing?	Possible Abnormal Findings
Scoliosis			
Kyphosis			
Ankylosing Spondylitis			
Spondylosis			
Spondylolithesis			

Pathology	Tests and Measures	What Is the Test and Measure Testing?	Possible Abnormal Findings
Compression Fractures			
Post-Surgical Spinal Procedures			
Thoracic Outlet Syndrome			
Arthritis			
Postural Dysfunctions			

Pathology	Tests and Measures	What Is the Test and Measure Testing?	Possible Abnormal Findings
Spinal Stenosis			
Sciatica			
Facet Dysfunctions			
Degenerative Disk Disease			
Nerve Compression			

Pathology	Tests and Measures	What Is the Test and Measure Testing?	Possible Abnormal Findings
Myelopathy			
Tumors			

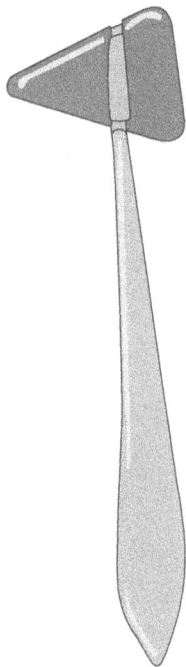

Reflex hammer

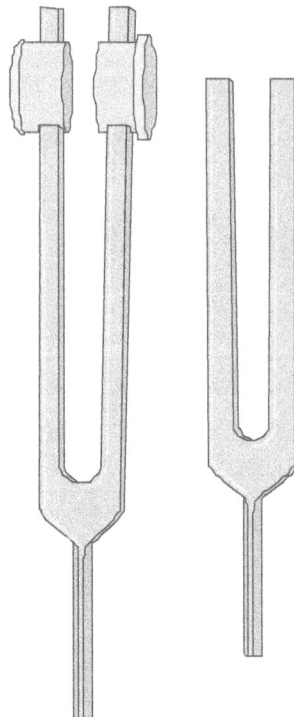

Tuning forks

INTERVENTIONS

Pathology	Intervention	Indication for Intervention	Goals for the Intervention	Contraindications of the Intervention	Settings for Intervention
	Ultrasound	Increase in pain, edema, and an increase in inflammatory response.	To decrease pain, decrease inflammatory response, and increase circulation to facilitate healing.	Pacemakers, cancer, plastic implants, pregnancy, joint cement, decreased sensation and mentation.	Will use a pulsed ultrasound 1 MHz at 2.0 w/cm² at 100% duty cycle × 10 minutes. Phonophoresis may be beneficial as well.
Ligamentous Strain					
Muscle Strain					
Ruptured/ Herniated Disk					
Scoliosis					

Pathology	Intervention	Indication for Intervention	Goals for the Intervention	Contraindications of the Intervention	Settings for Intervention
Kyphosis					
Ankylosing Spondylitis					
Spondylosis					
Spondylolithesis					
Compression Fractures					

Pathology	Intervention	Indication for Intervention	Goals for the Intervention	Contraindications of the Intervention	Settings for Intervention
Post-Surgical Spinal Procedures					
Thoracic Outlet Syndrome					
Arthritis					
Postural Dysfunctions					

Pathology	Intervention	Indication for Intervention	Goals for the Intervention	Contraindications of the Intervention	Settings for Intervention
Spinal Stenosis					
Sciatica					
Facet Dysfunctions					
Degenerative Disk Disease					
Compression					

Pathology	Intervention	Indication for Intervention	Goals for the Intervention	Contraindications of the Intervention	Settings for Intervention
Nerve					
Myelopathy					
Tumors					

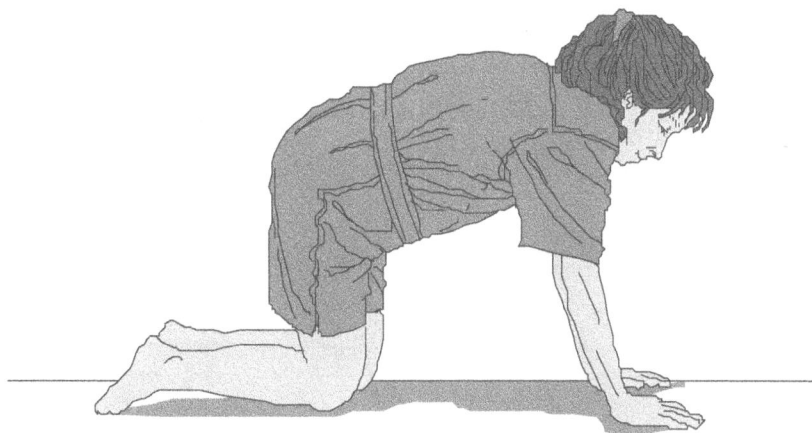

Arching back

Chapter 11

GAIT

Define the following terms:

1. Cadence

2. Step

3. Stride

4. Step Length

5. Stride Length

6. Gait Cycle

7. Base of Support

8. Center of Gravity

9. Single Stance

10. Double Stance

11. Nonsupport

Describe the different parts of the traditional gait cycle and the Rancho Los Amigos gait descriptions:

Traditional	**Rancho Los Amigos**
Heel Strike	Initial Contact
Foot Flat	Loading Response
Midstance	Terminal Stance
Heel Off	Preswing
Toe Off	Initial Swing
Acceleration	Midswing
Midswing	Terminal Swing
Deceleration	

For each of the phases of the gait cycle, describe what is happening at each of the joints:

	Traditional	**Rancho Los Amigos**
Hip		
Knee		
Ankle		
Spine		
Upper Extremities		

In each of the phases of the gait cycle, identify the muscles that are working eccentrically, concentrically, and isometrically:

	Concentric	Eccentric	Isometric
Heel Strike			
Foot Flat			
Midstance			
Heel Off			
Toe Off			
Acceleration			
Midswing			
Deceleration			

Fill out the following chart regarding possible gait abnormalities seen in each phase of the gait cycle:

	Abnormalities Observed
Heel Strike	
Foot Flat	
Midstance	
Heel Off	
Toe Off	
Acceleration	
Midswing	
Deceleration	

REFERENCES

Kendall, F., McCreary, E., Provance, P. G., Rodgers, M., & Romani, W. (2005). *Muscles: Testing and function with posture and pain.* New York, NY: LWW.

Komin, J. G., Wikaten, D. L., Isear, J. A., & Brader, H. (2002). *Special tests for orthopedic examination* (2nd ed.). Thorofare, NJ: SLACK.

Levangie, P. K., & Norkin, C. C. *Joint structure and function: A comprehensive analysis.* Philadelphia, PA: FA Davis.

Norkin, C. C., & White, D. J. *Measurement of joint motion: A guide to goniometry.* Philadelphia, PA: FA Davis.

Rothstein, J. M., Roy, S. H., & Wolf, S. L. (2005). *The rehabilitation specialist's handbook.* Philadelphia, PA: FA Davis.